# Birthing
## Naturally

'Pregnancy is a very important part of a woman's life. Considering the lifestyle being followed by couples these days, pregnancy definitely demands significant life changes. *Birthing Naturally* will motivate more mothers to stay fit and healthy during their pregnancy. This book will encourage mothers to prepare for a natural childbirth, thereby reducing the number of Caesarean-section deliveries in our country.'—Satyendar Jain, minister of health, industries, PWD, power, home and urban development, Delhi government

# Birthing Naturally

## Your Guide to a Stress-free Pregnancy and Natural Childbirth

# Dr Mahima Bakshi

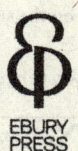

EBURY
PRESS

An imprint of Penguin Random House

EBURY PRESS

USA | Canada | UK | Ireland | Australia
New Zealand | India | South Africa | China | Singapore

Ebury Press is part of the Penguin Random House group of companies
whose addresses can be found at global.penguinrandomhouse.com

Published by Penguin Random House India Pvt. Ltd
4th Floor, Capital Tower 1, MG Road,
Gurugram 122 002, Haryana, India

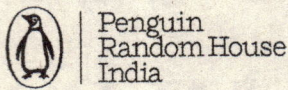

Penguin
Random House
India

First published in Ebury Press by Penguin Random House India 2018

10 9 8 7 6 5 4 3 2

ISBN 9780143441809

Typeset in Sabon by Manipal Digital Systems, Manipal

Printed at Repro India Limited

www.penguin.co.in

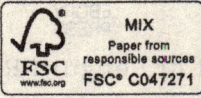

This is a legitimate digitally printed version of the book and therefore might not
have certain extra finishing on the cover.

# Contents

# Contents

# Foreword

We are all aware of the physical changes that a woman's body undergoes during pregnancy. Improper posture, reduced muscle strength, muscle spasms, low back pain, sacroiliac joint dysfunction and nerve irritation are common problems that accompany the physiological and anatomical changes. Good care during pregnancy is not only important for the health of the mother but also for the development of the growing foetus.

In today's fast-paced and health-conscious world, many women continue their exercise regimen even after pregnancy while others begin exercising during this period to improve their health and quality of life.

Every pregnancy is different and it is very important that every pregnant woman is taken care of adequately. So with an increasing demand for professional fitness service comes an opportunity for physiotherapists as they are well aware of the human anatomy and physiology and the changes that occur in the body during and after pregnancy. Physiotherapy during pregnancy can be useful for remedying common discomforts and musculoskeletal conditions, if any, and enhance the body's ability to have a smooth pregnancy and natural childbirth.

I truly believe that *Birthing Naturally* by Mahima Bakshi will provide physiotherapists with all the information required to assess, treat and educate women, while administering effective and safe exercises.

Together with a multidisciplinary approach, we can envision a world where every pregnant woman receives quality care during pregnancy and childbirth.

*With every child, a mother is born.*

Dr Ali Irani
President, Indian Association of Physiotherapists

# Introduction

Pregnancy is a beautiful phase of womanhood; unfortunately, many also fear the changes that accompany it—sometimes physical, sometimes emotional and sometimes both. Nausea, morning sickness, weight gain, labour pain, or the constant loss of sleep is symptomatic of this phase.

To deal with these various issues, one approaches a host of medical professionals—obstetricians, paediatricians, among others. But who does one approach for pregnancy wellness? During the last five years of my practice into mother and child wellness, which focuses on prenatal, perinatal, postnatal and lactation support, I have realized that many women still don't know how to take care of themselves during pregnancy. They choose to suffer silently rather than asking someone for help even though their problems can be solved with just a little bit of care and knowledge.

Every woman is different and so is every pregnancy. Seeking an expert's advice on pregnancy wellness will help you know about the dos and don'ts of this phase.

But an obstetrician might not be able to attend to all your queries due to her busy schedule and emergencies in the operating theatre; the Internet is not the best place to look for answers either. A more advisable idea is to know the basics yourself so that your pregnancy and labour is smoother and more comfortable.

Having conducted workshops on preconception, prenatal exercise, childbirth preparation, lactation and parenting at Fortis Escorts and Apollo Cradle India, I have discovered that many pregnant women don't have a guided support system to meet their emotional needs and to take care of their physical changes. Every woman wants her pregnancy to be hiccup-free, but few get the guidance to see the phase through as desired. This realization is what has given me the impetus to write a book that will help women who cannot access my sessions or that of an antenatal therapist's.

As a wellness consultant for women and children, the most gratifying parts of my job are to hold newborns in my arms during my daily rounds, and to help new mothers establish a successful breastfeeding routine. I had known since childhood that I wanted to help women out during their pregnancies, gift their babies a healthy and fit life. But ensuring good health begins from the preconception stage. Therefore, I coach women right from this stage to ensure wellness not just for themselves but also for their future babies.

A woman's body is made in such a way that it opens up naturally to bring forth a new life. But many Caesarean sections are due to a lack of preparation on the part of the mothers-to-be and not necessarily because of the nature of their pregnancies. Many women can't push due to lack of stamina; or they go through a prolonged labour spell as the cervical dilation is slow, or are unable to tolerate the pain and remain stiff.

This book is my humble attempt to help you prepare yourself for natural birthing; to equip you with all the tools and techniques that will make your experience easier and more comfortable. Please remember that till the last minute there is always the risk of having a Caesarean lest any medical conditions arise that might put your or the baby's safety in jeopardy. So prepare yourself and trust the judgement of your obstetrician.

As you enter your pregnancy, you will experience many changes, and as you progress in this phase, you will feel the need to constantly seek physical and emotional support. This book will help you as a guide, a friend and as an antenatal caregiver till you become a mother. I will guide you on the wellness of your mind, body and soul for each trimester of your pregnancy, preparing you and your partner for natural birthing.

So let the journey begin.

# Natural Childbirth

First, I need you to understand why natural childbirth is extremely important. The most important reason is to expose your baby to the microbiomes that are present in your vagina. Microbiomes are natural bacteria that are present in the human body. They help in strengthening the immune system. They are found in our skin, intestines, vagina and other parts of the body. Any shift in the natural levels of our microbiomes can lead to dysbiosis, which can in turn lead to many infections, diseases and even hormonal imbalance. Your baby will lose out on these microbiomes in a Caesarean birth, which will increase the risk of her developing infections later on.

Also, early breastfeeding will strengthen your baby's immunity. The initial milk, colostrum, is rich in antibodies and is a must for the baby. It's important to establish a successful breastfeeding relation between the mother and her baby. The first few hours are especially significant. The golden time is the first one hour after delivery. The baby must start breastfeeding within an hour of being born.

Also, early and frequent breastfeeding helps in enhancing milk production. If breastfeeding is delayed, it can lead to breast engorgement, which further hampers breastfeeding and can reduce milk production.

Now in case of a Caesarean section, the baby is not exposed to the microbiomes in the vagina. Anaesthesia and restriction of movement post the C-section makes it difficult for the mother to feed her baby. She has to be careful about her stitches as well and might be given a longer dose of antibiotics than someone who's given birth naturally. Many antibiotics are also given after a C-section to prevent infections in the stitches, which further kill the microbiomes in the body. This in turn reduces the immunity of the baby and the mother even more. Some contents of the antibiotics can transfer through breast milk, which means even the antibodies can get affected. Also, as early breastfeeding is difficult to establish after a C-section, the golden period is missed and breastfeeding gets delayed in most cases. Post the C-section, the mother is put on IV fluids for a while and gradually allowed an oral liquid diet, followed by a soft diet and proper food on the third day. A woman who has given birth naturally can have proper food on the same day of her delivery. Of course, a natural childbirth is exhausting and the mother requires rest and sleep, but she can take care of her baby as well.

A C-section, like all other types of surgeries, has side effects—excessive blood loss, damage to any surrounding vessel or structures in the body, weakened muscles and a long road to recovery. Pain in the stitches after a C-section can lead to irritability and lack of sleep, which can make you more vulnerable to depression. That's one reason why postnatal depression is more commonly found in women who have undergone a C-section. A study conducted by P.M. Boyce and A.L. Todd looked at the increased risk of postnatal depression after an emergency Caesarean section. The study concluded that, 'When compared with women having spontaneous vaginal or forceps deliveries, those having an emergency Caesarean section had more than six times the risk of developing postnatal depression three months postpartum. Special attention to this group appears warranted.'[1]

A natural vaginal delivery can be assisted if the labour is very exhausting for the mother or if the baby's head is not coming out properly. Your obstetrician-gynaecologist (ob–gyn) might decide to go for an assisted natural vaginal delivery. There are two types of assisted natural vaginal deliveries—forceps assistance and the vacuum-suction method. The natural vaginal delivery is assisted by the use of forceps or a vacuum suction to help the expulsion of the baby's head through the vagina. The rest of the body then follows. But eventually, it is the safety of the mother and the baby that is of paramount importance. And if your ob–gyn feels that none of the above ways are working, she can convert the labour into an emergency section to get the baby out immediately. This could happen in case of non-progressive labour—where your labour is not progressing from one stage to another for many hours; or if your baby's heart rate drops; or if there is an excessive drop or rise in your blood pressure during labour; or if the baby passes meconium, which is excreta expelled into the amniotic fluid, inside. Meconium can be ingested and could be fatal. Also, in situations where the size of the baby's head and the mother's pelvic size is not in sync to allow easy passage; or if the baby's head is not down (vertex down position), a planned C-section might be done. Also, in case of twins or triplets, the possibility of a Caesarean is always higher. In case the baby needs to be born prematurely when it is not fully developed, a Caesarean is a safer option.

But thanks to the rise in couples wanting to get educated about childbirth, there has been a trend of antenatal classes being conducted in almost all big hospitals and maternity centres. This has also led to an increase in the number of couples wanting to go for a natural birth instead of a C-section unless medically advised. But a lot of patients opt for C-sections to avoid the stress of a natural delivery, which has led to a surge in such surgeries over the past few years.

Some doctors perform 'mahurat deliveries' if a couple wants one. In some hospitals, the cost of a natural delivery and a Caesarean can vary, underlying some commercial purpose, but it is mostly the same for both everywhere. Also, a planned Caesarean is convenient for doctors rather than rushing at night for a natural childbirth. The practice can vary from doctor to doctor.

Anything that is natural will always be safe. Thanks to a quicker recovery after natural childbirth, your baby too will feel more secure as she will get to be with you immediately. You too can move around soon after your delivery. In fact, you are expected to visit the washroom to empty your bladder after giving birth. On the contrary,

C-section mothers' movements are restricted for twenty-four hours after the surgery. It could also depend how early or late your doctor allows you to move.

So it is important that you understand the benefits of a natural childbirth over a C-section before making a decision. You can join antenatal classes that will help you prepare your body for a natural childbirth. Breathing exercises, yoga and a balanced diet followed during pregnancy are essential.

You could either go for regular classes or learn the exercises and do some basic ones at home daily. In fact, take your partner as well for these classes and ask them to sit with you at home for the breathing exercises and yoga. It will not only help you stay motivated but might make your partner health conscious as well. Staying fit and eating healthy is your responsibility as a parent. So ensure that your partner too follows it along with you. Wouldn't you want your baby to be healthy right from the beginning? Think about how you, as a parent, play an important role in gifting fitness and good health to your baby.

You can clear all your doubts about a natural childbirth during your antenatal classes, or talk to your ob–gyn. You must get rid of the fear of a natural childbirth. Take as much counselling as required to help yourself get ready. Read as many books as you can to understand the positive aspects of a natural childbirth. Understand the techniques that will make natural childbirth easier for you.

Staying positive is very important. Don't let any negativity—others' unpleasant experiences of natural childbirth—affect you. Tell yourself the power to deliver naturally lies within you. Do your best to prepare for a natural childbirth. Remember, you have to make yourself confident to deliver naturally.

You can also opt for epidural anaesthesia to make natural childbirth less painful, if at all you feel you might need it.

It is easier to put the responsibility of doing a natural delivery on your ob–gyn, but it actually depends on you and your body. Urban women living in metropolitan cities and working in nine-to-five jobs need to understand that their current lifestyle increases the risk for complications during pregnancy and labour. Even the fertility rate is affected by one's lifestyle. You must prepare for a natural delivery that is easier and shorter in duration instead of blaming the ob–gyn for a C-section.

Discuss with your antenatal therapist if you want to have a natural birth and the effort needed for it. Once you cross thirty-seven weeks, sit with your birth coach and your partner and make a birth plan. Share it with your ob–gyn and discuss how ready you are to cope with her at each stage of your labour. Support from your partner at this stage is crucial. Your ob–gyn will back your birth plan as long as the baby is safe. You must have faith in her. However, if any risk is involved, or in cases where a natural delivery is not possible, then let her take a call. Believe in her; she will do the best for you and your baby.

Also, in case of a C-section, don't lose heart. You prepared for it and the preparation has benefitted you in many other ways. Your body will recover faster; you will feel more fit and active; your baby has benefitted from your prenatal yoga and exercises; you will be able to breastfeed with less pain in your back and neck as your muscles have been trained.

in many other ways. Your body will recover faster, you will feel more fit and active; your baby has benefited from your prenatal yoga and exercises, you will be able to breastfeed with less pain in your back and neck as your muscles have been trained.

# 2

# The ABC of Pregnancy

Pregnancy is a long journey to receive your little one in your arms. Your body will undergo many changes in these nine months and for a few months after your delivery. My attempt is to guide you on these changes and teach you ways to cope with them in each trimester so that your journey is comfortable and fearless. Knowledge is power, but having the right kind of knowledge is also equally important.

The nine months of gestation are divided into three phases known as trimesters.

- First trimester—one–three months.
- Second trimester—four–six months.
- Third trimester—seven–nine months.

Of all the phases, the third trimester is the most crucial one as labour preparation is mainly done during this time. As a part of this preparation, a couple learns how labour begins, its signs, and the partner's role during it as well as techniques to make the experience easier. These topics are generally covered in childbirth preparation classes or 'antenatal classes'. Although the third trimester is technically the last phase of gestation, the three months following delivery—also known as the fourth trimester—are equally important for keeping yourself healthy and fit. Generally, new mothers tend to ignore their health after having the baby as a new member in the family takes away all the attention.

## Weight Gain in Pregnancy

One of the most frequently asked questions during pregnancy is how soon a mother can shed weight after delivery.

But first let's tackle how you gain weight during pregnancy. And how to gain the right amount of weight that will make it less difficult to shed it off later. Most women with extra weight post-delivery are the ones who have gained excessively in unwanted areas during pregnancy. Some gain is natural but piling on unnecessary extra kilos can be avoided with a safe fitness routine. But is it safe for every woman and every kind of pregnancy?

The average weight gain during pregnancy is around 15 kg. Many of my patients ask me how much weight they need to gain, or remain worried that they are not gaining enough or gaining too much. There is no 'ideal weight gain' during pregnancy. If you are not gaining enough weight, visit your ob–gyn, who will help keep a close check on your baby and its growth. The doctor will see if your baby is gaining weight and growing as she is supposed to in conjunction with the number of weeks of your pregnancy. These regular examinations are conducted during your antenatal visits and helps in keeping track of your ultrasound reports as well.

It is important to eat right during this time. Therefore, it is advisable that you consult a dietitian with a sound knowledge of pregnancy nutrition. I have had so many cases of pregnant mothers telling me that they have already gained 10 kg early on in their second trimester. It is important to not exceed the weight gain limit—the threshold of which depends on your preconception weight. If you were underweight before you conceived, then you might put on up to 18 kg. Regular check-ups will ensure that the baby gains weight properly too. But if you were already overweight at the preconception stage, then you may put on up to 10 kg. However, if you were obese, then your ob–gyn will probably not want you to put on more than 5 kg.

Excessive weight gain can make you vulnerable to developing gestational diabetes and hypertension, which could pose a higher risk to the baby's growth and birth. So you need to keep a track of your weight gain to prevent such conditions from arising and to avoid having a C-section.

Gestational hypertension, also referred to as pregnancy-induced hypertension (PIH), is a condition characterized by high blood pressure during pregnancy. Hypertension during pregnancy affects around 6–8 per cent of women.

There are three common types of high blood pressure problems during pregnancy:

**Chronic Hypertension**—Women who have high blood pressure (over 140/90) before pregnancy, early in pregnancy (before twenty weeks), or those who continue having it after delivery.

**Gestational Hypertension**—High blood pressure that develops after the twentieth week and goes away after delivery.

**Pre-eclampsia**—Both chronic hypertension and gestational hypertension can lead to this severe condition after the twentieth week.

Symptoms include high blood pressure and protein in the urine. This can lead to serious complications for both the mother and the baby if not treated quickly.

Hypertension can prevent the placenta from getting enough blood. If the placenta doesn't get enough blood, your baby will get less oxygen and food. This can result in low birth weight. Most women can still deliver a healthy baby if hypertension is detected and treated early on.[2]

Some contributing factors to high blood pressure can be controlled, while others cannot. Follow your doctor's instruction about diet and exercise. Some ways in which you can prevent gestational hypertension are:

- Use salt only as needed for taste.
- Drink at least eight glasses of water every day.
- Increase the amount of protein you take in and decrease the amount of fried food and junk food consumed.

- Get enough rest.
- Exercise regularly.
- Elevate your feet several times during the day.
- Avoid beverages containing caffeine.

The presence of gestational diabetes during pregnancy can adversely affect both you and your baby's health. You must not neglect this area to ensure the safety of your baby. If you have a family history of diabetes, you have to tell your ob–gyn about it. She will check with you in case you were already suffering from diabetes even before conception.

A poor lifestyle can always put anyone at a high risk for diabetes. Even schoolchildren nowadays are diagnosed with diabetes. This is one area that should not be neglected at any age. You don't want your baby to be put at a high risk for developing diabetes later. Also, gestational diabetes can make the baby overweight, which can further lead to complications during delivery as the baby's head might not be in proportion to your pelvic size. You will read more about the effects of gestational diabetes on your baby later in this book.

Stay fit and healthy throughout pregnancy by eating right and exercising under expert guidance to prevent complications such as gestational diabetes and hypertension.

## The Antenatal Period

The antenatal (before birth) period is a vital time during pregnancy. It is a well-recognized fact that good antenatal care improves maternal, perinatal and neonatal outcomes. Many women will progress through pregnancy in an uncomplicated manner and deliver a healthy infant with little medical intervention, but a significant number will develop medical or foetal complications.

The present situation is alarming enough for us to identify women at a higher risk of developing such complications during pregnancy. Therefore, the role that a specialist plays in ensuring a smooth pregnancy without any bumps has become an imperative. The purpose of antenatal care is to help a woman make the right choices for pregnancy care, opt for the right delivery place, identify risks involved, and be aware about her pregnancy and childbirth.

## History of Antenatal Care

Scottish physician and obstetrician J.W. Ballantyne mentions in his book *Expectant Motherhood*:

India was the subject of various foreign influences and powers such as the Portuguese, the French, and most notably the British (339 years) till India won its independence from Britain in 1947 and became a free democratic country. After World War II, India, like other developing countries, underwent an era of immense population growth. This was due to a slightly lower birth rate and a significant reduction in death rate. Changes in maternity care policies and practices since 1948 have resulted in a huge growth in the number of hospital deliveries and the wider medicalization of birth.[3]

## Health Statistics

A survey on economic inequalities in maternal healthcare found that:

> The percentage of women in India who had an unmet need for family planning is 21 per cent. Seventy-five per cent of women have one visit covered by insurance for antenatal visits. Fifty per cent of women have at least four antenatal visits covered by their insurance. Sixty-seven per cent of women in India have their births attended by a skilled medical professional. In 2015, India's maternal mortality was 174 per 100,000 live births. In 2005, it was estimated that the maternal mortality ratio in India was sixteen times higher than that of Russia, ten times that of China and four times higher than Brazil. Among the developing countries, India contributes to the largest amount of births in the world a year, around 27 million. Unfortunately, India also accounts for 20 per cent of global maternal deaths in a year.[4]

## Prenatal Check-ups in Each Trimester

The Government of India mandates every pregnant woman should have access to antenatal care and at least a minimum of five such visits. The aim of every check-up during pregnancy is to ensure the well-being of both mother and child. If any risk factor is identified in time, it can be managed to ensure a safe pregnancy and childbirth.

The following will help you plan your visit to the doctor better:

- Have an early check-up with your doctor. This is the time when guidance on starting supplementation like folic acid, iron and so on are given. Also, other risk factors are assessed and previous history of any medical problem is taken into account.

- High-risk factors, such as maternal age (teenage or elderly), weight (undernourished or obese), risk of diabetes or pre-eclampsia in pregnancy must be checked. This is done by analysing the history of any maternal medical or surgical problems, and any previous pregnancies and their outcomes. Any medication, if required for nausea and vomiting, is generally started now.

- By the tenth week of pregnancy, visit your doctor to get information about your baby's growth, the importance of diet and nutrition, exercises in the antenatal period and the various tests that need to be done to screen for infections, anaemia and foetal well-being.

- A discussion of a pregnancy plan, place of delivery and importance of breastfeeding is essential.

- Also, by this visit the expecting mother's urine test for infection and proteinuria, blood test for checking the blood group, Rh typing, haemoglobin, HIV, HBsAg, rubella antibodies, syphilis should be done. At least one ultrasound needs to be done by this time. This is to confirm foetal viability, number and accurately date the pregnancy and rule out any early structural abnormalities.

- An ultrasound is essential between eleven to fourteen weeks when the length and the neck thickness need to be measured. This is then coupled with a blood test for screening of Down's Syndrome. If this test is negative, it means that risk of the foetus having chromosomal anomalies is low. If it is positive, additional tests like non-invasive blood tests or invasive tests have to be done to rule out the presence of any chromosomal anomaly.

- The next visit is by the sixteenth week when the urine needs to be checked for protein and bacteria. It is essential to check your blood pressure and you will be reassessed for high-risk factors. The patient is counselled about the right diet, balanced with proteins, carbohydrates and fats. If anaemia is identified, iron supplementation is started.

- A detailed ultrasound at around twenty weeks can be done to check for any significant abnormalities in the baby.

- The next appointment is by the twenty-fifth to twenty-sixth week, at which point foetal growth and well-being is assessed along with BP and proteinuria check. Blood sugar by the glucose tolerance test is checked. By this time, the expecting mother should decide the place and the hospital for delivery. Air travel is permitted up to thirty weeks as supported by the treating obstetrician. So if you're planning on having your baby outside the city that you reside in, plan well in advance. A hospital well equipped with all the necessary care facilities for the mother and the baby should be chosen.

- The twenty-eighth week marks the beginning of the third trimester of pregnancy. In this stage, haemoglobin is rechecked, anti D is given for Rh negative woman, and BP and proteinuria is checked again. The next visit is in the thirty-first week to reassess maternal BP, foetal growth and maternal proteinuria.

- In the thirty-sixth week, signs of labour and the plan for delivery are discussed. The mother is checked for BP, proteinuria, foetal position. Delivery, maternal and baby care after delivery, breastfeeding, vaccination of the baby, contraception post-delivery, etc., are discussed with the mother.

- In the thirty-eighth week, BP, foetal growth is rechecked. Reassurance from the team of doctors helps alleviate anxiety.

- If the mother has not yet delivered, the next visit is in the fortieth week to reassess BP, growth, and also to discuss post-dated pregnancy and the need for inducing labour if it continues after forty-one weeks.

- During the antenatal period, a primigravida, that is a women who is pregnant for the first time, needs to have about ten visits, and someone who has had a normal pregnancy before needs around seven visits for adequate care.

## Estimating the Due Date

- For accurate estimation of the due date, a maternal history of the menstrual cycle needs to be taken. The mother's last menstrual period (LMP) is the most important information that needs to be obtained. The regularity, duration and frequency of the cycle need to be ascertained properly.

- According to Naegele's rule, the due date is nine months and seven days after the LMP. The LMP is calculated from the first day of the last menstrual period when the mother had regular periods (twenty-eight days +/- seven days).

- If the expecting mother doesn't remember her last period, or has had irregular cycles, then she needs to get an early dating ultrasound that will predict the probable due date.

- The due date calculated by history is correlated with an ultrasound. The difference should be less than one week. If there is a discrepancy, then the due date by an early ultrasound (less than ten weeks) will help estimate the correct date.

- This calculation is important to facilitate detection of any growth delay. In cases where pregnancy is prolonged beyond forty weeks, it is helpful to decide on the date of induction of labour. Imagine making a batch of popcorn. Most of the kernels pop during a few noisy moments. But there are lots of early and late poppers too. All the popped kernels are perfect, but each needs a slightly different amount of time to be fully cooked. The same is true for babies.

- Though you and your ob–gyn might calculate a due date forty weeks from the first day of your last period, keep in mind that only about 5 per cent of babies arrive on their due dates. Many factors make due dates difficult to pin down. For example, the formula described above assumes a woman has a twenty-eight-day cycle and ovulates on the fourteenth day, which isn't true for many others. And some babies just take more or less than forty weeks to be ready for the outside world.

## How Can One Track a Baby's Growth According to Each Trimester?

- In the first twenty weeks, growth is checked through ultrasounds. By the second trimester, the uterus starts becoming big enough to be checked by an examination of the abdomen. The baby's growth is checked routinely at every visit by analysing the height and girth of the uterus, also called symphysiofundal height and girth.
- After twenty-four weeks, the symphysiofundal height is checked. This can help determine if further assessment is required.
- Ultrasound studies for foetal size and blood flow through uterine and umbilical arteries can help determine if the baby's growth is normal, slow or fast in accordance with growth charts. If there is a growth lag, additional protein and micronutrients in the diet and rest for a working woman are advised. If a rise in blood pressure or a medical condition is detected, then necessary intervention is advised and the mother is called at frequent intervals for clinical and ultrasound examinations.

## Summary of Recommendations

The World Health Organization's (WHO) recommendations on antenatal care for a positive pregnancy experience states:

A minimum of nine visits are recommended to improve antenatal care and baby outcome. The Government of India recommends a minimum of three sonographies—one at twelve weeks and one at nineteen weeks (early ultrasound)—for pregnant women to estimate the gestational age, improve detection of foetal anomalies and multiple pregnancies, and the third one at around thirty weeks to ensure foetal well-being. However, at times, additional scans are recommended to optimize the perinatal outcome. A good communication between the pregnant woman and her team of doctors and nurses helps to build up a smooth relationship and faith and this certainly eases out problems during the antenatal period and delivery.

3

# The First Trimester

As your pregnancy starts, you enter your first trimester. I have heard so many interesting stories about how patients found out that they were pregnant—some discovered it in their second month of pregnancy while some who had desperately longed for a baby kept testing their urine whenever they missed their periods.

In this chapter I will guide you through the kind of changes your body undergoes in the first three months of conception.

## The Magic of Pregnancy

The hormonal changes in your body caused by pregnancy can take you for a ride. The first trimester could show symptoms like nausea, vomiting, dizziness, hyperacidity, irritated mood, inability to sleep properly at night or excessive sleepiness. So the entire first trimester will mostly be spent in letting your body understand these changes and be able to cope with them later. Avoid exertion if you feel tired; don't force yourself to do something if you are not in the mood for it. I personally believe that no heavy exercises should be done during this phase. Your baby is yet to be formed, let Mother Nature do her work. Deal with this phase with care. If you have been going to the gym before conceiving, it is advisable to take a break from it. If any signs of bleeding or spotting occur in this phase, please inform your doctor immediately. No medication should be taken without the approval of your obstetrician.

If you are a working woman, you may continue going to work but if the nausea and vomiting leaves you drained, then take a few days off and rest under the medical advice of your obstetrician. Remember, stress can aggravate these signs and can make the first trimester even more difficult for you. It is very important to be calm and relaxed. Both work-related and family-related stress can worsen your nausea and vomiting, especially if it's an unplanned pregnancy. Hence, you must make meditation a part of your regular routine, especially during this phase.

## Meditation

Meditation is very effective in pregnancy to help you cope with first trimester changes.

Find the most comfortable corner of your home, one that is well-ventilated and where no one will disturb you. Dim the lights and make sure you have enough fresh air flowing in.

Gradually, let your eyes close and observe your breathing pattern. Breathe in through your nose and breathe out through your mouth (like blowing off a candle). Concentrate on your breathing. And let a rhythm form. Remember, it should be a fluidic rhythm.

Now while you breathe, imagine two balls, one red and the other blue. While you inhale, your mind tries to pull the blue ball towards you. It represents positive energy. And while you exhale, try to push away the red ball as it represents negative energy. With each breath you take, teach your body to relax. Place your hands on your abdomen and stick it out when you inhale and suck it in when you exhale. This will ensure deeper breathing and will relax your body further.

Meditation can be done at any time of the day. In fact, it is good to begin your day with lots of positive energy for yourself and your baby. You could even repeat it at work or even after coming back home in the evenings. It can really help you relieve all that work-related stress. Remember, the more frequently you do it throughout the day, the better you will feel. During the breathing exercise, try to feel an inner happiness and prepare yourself to gradually enjoy your way to motherhood. This exercise can also be done at bedtime with the lights turned off to induce better sleep.

## Music Therapy

For even better results I suggest combining meditation and music together. There are various tracks that are designed especially for pregnancy. Various researches have proven that pregnancy music tracks are very beneficial, not only in relaxing the mother but also in the better sensory development of the baby. I recommend all my patients to listen to 'Mozart for pregnancy' tracks; but there are many others also available online. Mozart's music has been proven to be very effective in stage one to ease labour when combined with other exercises and positioning. There are certain birthing positions that help in easing labour during stage one. As you read further, you will get to know the various stages of labour and the birthing positions that can help you.

## Are You Sick of Morning Sickness?

Try to check if there is any specific type of smell or fragrance that makes you nauseated. For some of you, it could even be the smell of your regular toothpaste or your favourite perfume or deodorant. Even your partner's perfume! So please try to identify that smell and get rid of it immediately. Also, check all your food. Sometimes the aroma of any food or vegetable or fruit can make you nauseated. Many of my patients complain feeling nauseated after having eggs. A red apple can also make you feel sick. So in case you're suffering from acidity, simply swap your red apple with a golden or green one. Apple is a very rich source of all the essential vitamins, iron and antioxidants. Do not skip eating it during pregnancy.

## KNOW YOUR NOSE

- If you can't stand the smell inside a kitchen or a restaurant, leave immediately.
- Frequently open your kitchen windows or run the exhaust fan.
- Wash your clothes more often than usual, since fibres tend to hold on to odours. Use unscented detergent and softener.
- Switch to unscented or mildly scented toiletries.
- Get your partners to wash up, change their clothes, and brush their teeth after meals.
- Avoid people who are smoking.
- Try to surround yourself with scents that make you feel better. Mint, lemon, ginger and cinnamon are more likely to be soothing.

## Distraction Therapy

Distraction therapy can be very beneficial in coping with pregnancy nausea. It will help you stay calm and reduce acidic production. You may read magazines or books or watch your favourite shows at the onset of nausea. Talking to friends can also serve as a good distraction. Remember, pregnancy is not an illness. It can be a smooth journey with concerned measures and guidelines by an expert.

You also need a lot of rest during this stage. Most of you will start putting on weight. Some may not able to eat well due to constant vomiting or nausea and might stay the same or even lose a bit of weight. You don't have to panic. Remember, there are medications available for managing the vomiting or severe nausea. But take these only after consulting your obstetrician. It's best to use natural techniques. Mind and soul exercises are very beneficial and should be done regularly along with music therapy for better results.

Eat at regular intervals; an empty stomach might cause problems. You should have small and light meals every two hours. Keep wholegrain cookies in your purse always. Remember to munch on something every two hours even when you are working and at office. You can set reminders on your phone for this. Eating on time helps in reducing acidity or nausea to some extent. Avoid eating food outside. Stick to homemade food to prevent a stomach infection. Spicy or oily food can lead to some discomfort or indigestion—they are better avoided. Ginger and mint also help in controlling nausea and indigestion. Try adding some to your food while cooking. You can also drink mint water instead of plain water a couple of times every day. Try to drink fresh tender coconut water daily. It's a rich source of multivitamins, which will balance the loss due to vomiting or nausea. Also, the vitamins help in the better growth of your baby. Supplements can also be taken under the guidance of your obstetrician. Remember to drink plenty of fluids.

You may experience some mood swings or feel cranky at times. It could be due to the changes happening in your body. Don't worry; your body is gradually trying to adapt to the changes and as the pregnancy progresses, your journey will get smoother. Just tell yourself repeatedly to stay calm with the various techniques that I have mentioned earlier. Remember, the more you practise them, the calmer you will feel.

## Common Changes You Need to Be Prepared for in Your First Trimester

### Tender or Swollen Breasts

The initial hormonal changes can make your breasts tender or too sensitive. You may experience discomfort while sleeping or wearing a bra. However, it will gradually decrease as your body gets used to these changes.

Tip—Avoid wearing a padded bra; wear non-padded, non-underwired ones.

### Nausea or Vomiting

Morning sickness, as mentioned initially, is also a usual feature for some women in their first trimester. Consult your ob–gyn if it affects your daily routine too much. You might be put on medication. This feeling should gradually go away in the second trimester.

Tip—Have a banana or Chamomile tea or cold almond milk.

### Increased Urination

You may have frequent urination than in your non-pregnant state.

Tip—Keep yourself well hydrated and do lots of Kegel exercises (explained in Chapter 4).

## Fatigue

You may feel like you get tired too easily. Don't worry, you should be feeling more active in your second trimester.

Tip—Take some rest or cat naps after your meals.

## Constipation or Loose Stool

You may experience severe constipation or loose motions in your first trimester. Some women could experience it from taking iron supplements. Discuss this with your ob–gyn. They might change your supplement if necessary.

Tip—Prunes for constipation; a lot of fluids in case of loose stools.

## Emotional Changes

The excitement of being pregnant will just take away all your other priorities for a while. This is especially true for those trying to conceive for a long time. Enjoy the feeling and cherish it.

However, if it's an unplanned pregnancy, you might feel stressed about continuing it. Talk to your ob–gyn or your partner. It will help you prepare mentally to continue the pregnancy.

Tip—Share the happiness and joy with your loved ones, it will make you happier!

## Diet in First Trimester

You might find it difficult to eat in case of morning sickness. But you shouldn't feel weak. So try to have small meals more frequently.

You should have a lot of fluids—coconut water and lemon water are especially good options. Cold milk, lassi, buttermilk are not bad either.

Try to have some curd if you cannot have a full meal. Have a lot of fruits.

Here is what your diet chart should look like:

6 a.m.—One glass of milk and some soaked nuts.

8 a.m.—Poha; upma; idli or cereals with a boiled egg.

10 a.m.— An apple or a banana.

12 p.m.—Coconut water

2 p.m.—One roti or one bowl of rice, subzi or daal, dahi, salad (lunch).

4 p.m.—Lemon water; lassi or buttermilk.

6 p.m.—Fruits (citrus ones).

8 p.m.—Chicken soup or broccoli soup with some brown rice and salad. You can also have one roti, daal, subzi and salad (dinner).

10 p.m.—A glass of cold milk.

## Exercise in First Trimester

I personally don't advise much exercising to my patients during this stage. I advise them to avoid heavy workouts. Breathing exercises are good. A little walking is fine to help your digestion. Just cope with the changes that are new for your body! Let your baby form safely.

## FIRST TRIMESTER

— Small six–eight meals per day.
— Meals should be very light.
— Have more fruits, khichdi, daal and curd.
— Drink a lot of fluids.
— Breathing exercises and meditation.
— Music therapy.

**4**

# The Second Trimester

As the fourth month begins, you enter your second trimester. Your body now understands the demands of your hormones and has mostly adapted to the changes. Symptoms like nausea and vomiting will gradually reduce and you will be able to enjoy eating now. So eat well during this phase and let your baby get enough nutrition. Also, if your condition is fine, this is a good time for you to start exercising. Remember, the healthier you eat, the better your baby grows and develops.

## Changes in the Second Trimester

### Breast Size Increases

This phase is marked by greater physical changes than your first trimester due to more hormonal differences. Your breasts will feel fuller or heavier.

Tip—Change your bra according to the increase in breast size.

## Growing Belly

As your uterus expands to give more space to your growing baby, you will now find your pants getting tighter and notice a small bump.

Tip—Wear loose, comfortable clothes or maternity pants and jeggings.

## Skin Changes

Some of you might notice dark patches developing on your face and neck while some might just enjoy a natural glow. This is very unpredictable.

Tip—Take care of your skin. Refer to Chapter 22 on skin care.

## Stretch Marks

As your skin stretches to accommodate the weight gain and your baby inside you, stretch marks will start appearing around your breasts and belly.

Tip—Keep your skin moisturized and eat a nutritious diet. Refer to Chapter 22.

## Baby Movements

This can start around the fourth or the fifth month. Initially, you will feel butterfly-like movements in your belly. They tend to get more pronounced in your third trimester. Enjoy the baby moving inside you, bond with her.

## Mood Swings

You will now experience emotional outbursts or an excessive urge to cry. You may also get irritated or angry too easily and for no visible reason. These moods are due to hormonal changes. You need not panic as it is very common.

Tip—Relaxation techniques and yoga help in staying calm.

# Are You Passing a Lot of Gas?

Are you passing more gas than usual? Nobody is as flatulent as a pregnant woman. Fortunately, while the same can't be said for those who work and live within hearing and sniffing distance of you, your baby is oblivious and impervious to your digestive distress. Snug and safe in the uterine cocoon that's protected on all sides by the impact-absorbing amniotic fluid, the baby is probably soothed by the bubbling and gurgling of your gastric sounds. It can make you feel quite uneasy, but do not try to hold the gas inside you, which can prove to be really discomforting. Release it no matter who is around. It's fine; people know you are pregnant.

The baby won't be happy, though, if the bloating, which often worsens late in the day and, yes, generally persists throughout pregnancy, prevents you from eating regularly and well. To cut down on the sounds and smells from down under and to make sure your nutritional intake doesn't suffer on account of your intestinal outbreak, take the following measures:

Stay Regular—Constipation is a common cause of gas and bloating. Take lots of fibre-rich food. Include fresh fruits and salads in your diet. Drink a lot of water. Check your supplementation with your ob–gyn.

**Small Meals**—Large meals just add to that bloated feeling. They also overload your digestive system, which isn't at its most efficient anyway during pregnancy. Instead of those two or three heavy meals, take six small meals.

**Don't Rush**—When you rush through meals or eat on the fly, you are bound to swallow as much as air as food. This captured air forms painful pockets of gas in your gut, which seek release the only way they know.

**Stay Calm**—Particularly during meals, tension and anxiety can cause you to swallow air, which can give you a full tank of gas. Taking a few deep breaths before meals may help relax you.

**Stay Away from Gas-Producing Food**—Your tummy will tell you what they are; they vary from person to person. Common items include onions, cabbage, fried food, sweets, carbonated beverages, beans, etc.

**Don't Take Anti-Gas Syrups**—Ask your practitioner before taking your usual anti-gas syrups. Hot water with lemon and Chamomile tea are safer options and helpful in relieving gas-like symptoms.

Also, staying in one position can aggravate the symptoms. You must move around. Walk around a bit and do antenatal yoga asanas (but not if bed rest is advised).

## Are You Eating Right?

The second phase of your pregnancy can be best enjoyed as it gradually progresses. Some of you might have put on a few kilos by now. Ideally it should be 1–2 kg but every pregnancy is different. You may put on 1–2 kg per month in this phase and around 1 kg every fifteen days in the third trimester. Eat healthy and check your weight every week; make a chart.

You should alter your diet according to the amount of weight you have gained. Of course, if you are already overweight or obese, I suggest you consult a dietitian and get a customized diet chart whether you are diabetic or not. Mostly, try to follow a four-part-meal method: proteins, simple carbohydrates, healthy fats, and fruits and vegetables.

Practise mindful eating—it is very important during pregnancy. It helps provide more nutrition to the baby, which is essential for its growth and development.

Here are some tips to help you practice eating with awareness: Eating is akin to a form of meditation and must be performed in a relaxed state of mind and without anyone disturbing you. Avoid talking while eating. Try to enjoy the taste of the bite and chew every morsel multiple times. This will better absorb nutrients. Remember, if you eat healthy and right, along with the right exercises, in your second and third trimester, then you are almost on the right track. However, some issues like gestational diabetes might demand a modification in your diet. So keep consulting your ob–gyn during your regular antenatal visits.

Here is how your healthy balanced diet should look during pregnancy:

On waking up:

- Light tea (with mint preferably) and biscuits; or a glass of cold milk and banana if nauseated or have acidity or morning sickness.

You can have any of the following for breakfast:

- Muesli/porridge with a few raisins, eight almonds, two walnuts and milk.
- One–two slices of multigrain toast, fresh fruits with yoghurt and nuts.
- Idli or poha or upma and fresh fruits and milk.
- Egg, bread and fruits.

Mid-morning (two–three hours after breakfast):

- Fresh vegetable juice; coconut water or lemon juice

Lunch:

- Two chapatis or a bowl of rice with a bowl of subzi, two bowls of daal or a piece of chicken or fish and curd.

Evening:

- A cup of milk or fruits.

Dinner (any one of the following):

- A bowl of salad.
- Sprouts or boiled chana with a carrot or two tomatoes and cucumber or lettuce or coriander.
- Soya; paneer; cooked vegetables and brown rice.
- Soup.
- A chapati or rice (second trimester).

Bedtime: A glass of milk.

As you are put on iron and calcium supplements, you need to ensure that you space out your supplements intake properly. Do not take your iron and calcium supplements together. Also, do not take your iron supplement along with milk. Have your calcium supplement with breakfast and the iron supplement after lunch around 4 p.m. if you are not drinking milk at 5 p.m.

Fat is also important for absorption of some vitamins. Good fats like omega-6 and omega-3 fatty acids are healthy.

Almonds, walnuts, soyabean are healthy food, so are jaggery, dates, prunes and chocolates. Avoid cakes and sweets like *halwas* and junk food and don't use too much ghee. You may use around one teaspoon throughout the day, which can be put in daal or applied a little on chapatis. We need some fat for the absorption of vitamin D, which is a fat-soluble vitamin. Other fat-soluble vitamins are A, E and K.

Use fresh fruits and vegetables. Sprouts, broccoli, fermented food like idli, dhokla, etc., act as an added source of B complex vitamins. Use coloured fruits and vegetables like oranges, etc. Avoid frozen chicken or fish. Iron is very important for the baby's brain development and for the mother as there is heavy loss of blood at the time of delivery. More iron means better oxygen-carrying capacity too. Junk food and items with preservatives can make you gain excess unhealthy fat; steer clear of them. Avoiding such food will also help you get back in shape early.

So every time you crave for munchies between your meals, here are some healthy options for you:

- Roasted murmure and flakes
- Roasted chana
- Almonds and walnuts
- Yoghurt
- Banana
- Brown bread vegetable sandwich
- Multigrain cookies
- Wholegrain roll
- Mini-meal soya nuggets or kebabs
- Pita pocket with hummus
- Idli chaat
- Bhel
- One serving of stir-fried veggies with rice
- Stuffed parantha

## Are You Drinking Enough Water?

If you don't drink sufficient water, you might get infections. And the administration of unnecessary medicinal drugs must be avoided during pregnancy. So prevent infections by increasing your daily intake of water. You must:

- Drink at least four litres daily.
- Start your day with a glass of water.
- Have a glass of water every hour.
- Carry a bottle with you always.
- Increase your intake of fresh fruits and salads as they have a high water content.
- Don't wait to get thirsty.
- Drink various forms of fluids like buttermilk or lemonade or coconut water or fresh juices, etc.

Plenty of water will also hydrate your skin and prevent stretch marks, adding more glow.

## Avoiding Water because of Frequent Visits to the Loo?

Drinking more water also means frequent urination. You must do Kegel exercises to strengthen your bladder muscles. How many of you actually think of returning your pelvic muscles and uterus as well as vaginal muscles back to their original shapes? Everyone thinks of their outward forms but internal structures also expand during pregnancy and labour; they too need care and attention.

Kegels will help you regain strength in the pelvic muscles, tighten the vaginal muscles and ease you back to enjoying sex after delivery.

## How Can One Perform Kegel Exercises?

Imagine that your bladder is full and you need to stop urine from passing. Contract the same set of muscles the way you would do in such a situation and count till five. Then gradually start contracting the bladder muscles— count one, two, three, four, five . . . while imagining an elevator going up the floors in a gradual manner. And then gradually relax your muscles just like the elevator would go down. Don't let go suddenly.

Kegels should be done throughout the first trimester too. This can be done even by non-pregnant women.

```
KEGEL—THE MAGIC EXERCISE

• Driving? Kegels at the traffic signal.
• Office? Kegels at the desk.
• Cooking? Kegels in the kitchen.
• Texting? Kegels while chatting.
• About to sleep? Do Kegels as you fall asleep.
```

You must do Kegels 100–200 times a day for it to be effective. The range might sound scary but once you start doing the exercise, it won't seem so daunting. It's an internal exercise and you can do it anywhere; you don't need a mat or a ball for it. You just need to make it a habit.

---

### SECOND TRIMESTER

— Follow the four-part-meal method. Include cereals, fruits, vegetables and sweets.
— Drink a lot of water.
— Add a lot of protein to your food.
— Do antenatal exercises.

— ...
— Do antenatal exercises.

5

# Antenatal Exercises

## Exercise the Right Way

A lot of pregnancy-related problems like gestational
diabetes, hypertension or thyroid dysfunction can be
prevented to an extent with antenatal exercises, which
is why I cannot stress on their importance enough. Also,
regular antenatal exercises help in reducing pain related
to varicose veins, swelling in the hands or feet, leg cramps
and even backaches.

You may enrol for antenatal sessions at your hospital,
if available, or find out a well-trained antenatal expert
in your area. It will help if they know your pregnancy
history or placenta position, so exercises can be suggested
accordingly. Remember, antenatal exercises should not be
learnt from any untrained person as it might harm your
baby if not done properly and an expert will know what
has to be kept in mind before deciding the exercises that are
safe for you. Also, the exercises may have to be changed or

stopped depending upon how your pregnancy progresses. After you have entered your second trimester, you must ask your ob–gyn if you can start exercising or not. Keep updating your antenatal expert with your reports.

There are numerous benefits of antenatal sessions and exercises:

- Help in regaining your confidence to deliver naturally according to your own potential.
- Prepare you to stay strong, calm and healthy.
- Help you and your baby to stay fit and healthy.
- Keep a check on your weight and help you get back in shape soon after delivery.
- Especially helpful for working mothers.

Listed below are the different forms of antenatal exercises:

## Breathing Exercises

These can be done even during the first trimester.

## Physio

Ensure strengthening of your muscles; helps in preventing pain.

## Antenatal Yoga

Helps in birthing naturally.

## Antenatal Aerobics

Build endurance in pushing during labour and recovering faster after birth. They also improve your breathing capacity, which generally reduces in the third trimester.

## Antenatal Pilates

Strengthen your core to ensure a faster recovery of your abdomen after birth.

## Couple Exercises

I personally promote couple exercises during pregnancy. They help in involving the partner equally in your pregnancy. You can ask them to take you out for maternity shopping as the baby bump appears. You can go out for dinner as you no longer feel nauseated and the antenatal exercises help in maintaining a healthy lifestyle. But do go only to hygienic restaurants. Now is a good time to socialize as well. Such interactions keep you emotionally and mentally healthy. Try to avoid discussions on negative accounts of pregnancies or deliveries. I always tell my patients to stay positive and only hear positive stories related to pregnancy. See a comedy or a romantic film rather than a horror or an action one. Do not have excess popcorn. It can lead to belching or indigestion or stomach infection. When out for a movie, keep moving your legs at frequent intervals.

## Exercise Time at Home

Here are some exercises that you could perform at home after checking with your ob–gyn. Also, meet an antenatal expert who will explain the right exercises for you. There are some exercises that might not be good for you considering your scan status. You must show your scan reports to an expert to be sure about the safety of your exercises.

**Ankle Exercises** (Can be started from the first trimester)

These exercises can be done in a lying position at home or while sitting in office or in a car or a cinema hall.

Stretch your legs away from your body and pull your toes towards yourself and then away (up/down).

In the same way, rotate your feet in clockwise/anticlockwise direction fifteen–twenty times each.

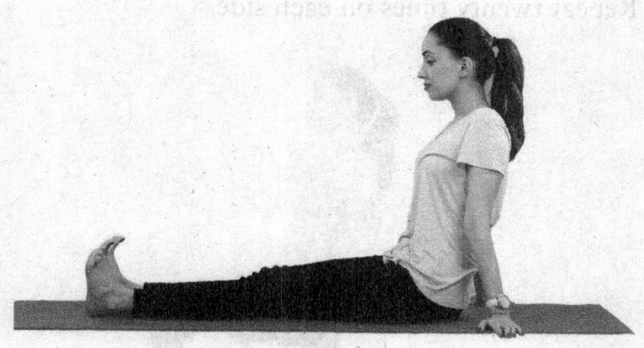

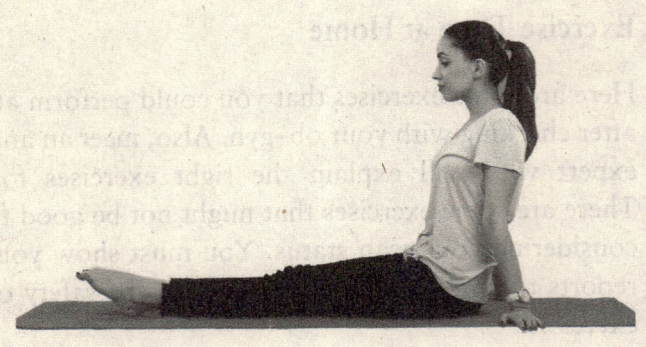

**Knee Exercises** (Can be started in the first trimester)

In a lying or sitting position, stretch your legs and press your knees downwards on to the bed or mat. Hold for five seconds and then relax. Repeat twenty times on each side.

In a sitting position on a chair in office, stretch your legs, bringing your feet upwards and pull your toes towards yourself. Hold for five seconds and then relax, while bringing your feet down with your knees bending. Repeat twenty times on each side.

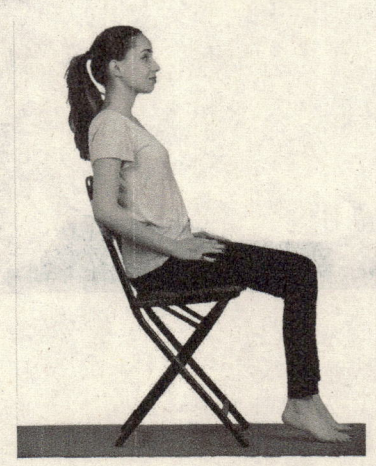

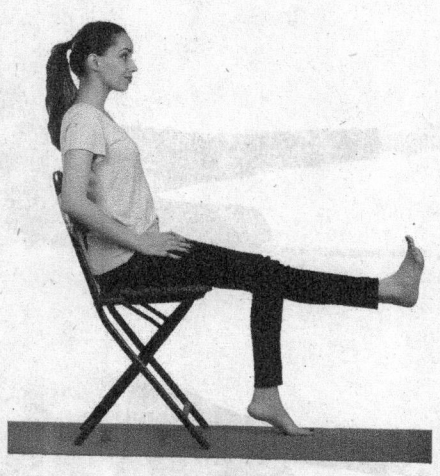

Knee-extension exercise on a chair

**Hip Exercises** (Can be started from first trimester)

In a sitting or lying position, do butt squeezes. Maintain each for five seconds and repeat twenty–thirty times.

While lying sideways, raise your leg upwards while keeping your knees straight. Hold for five seconds and then relax while you lower your leg. Repeat fifteen times on each side. Make sure you don't hold your breath at any point during any of these exercises. Learn your breathing technique from your antenatal expert for each exercise.

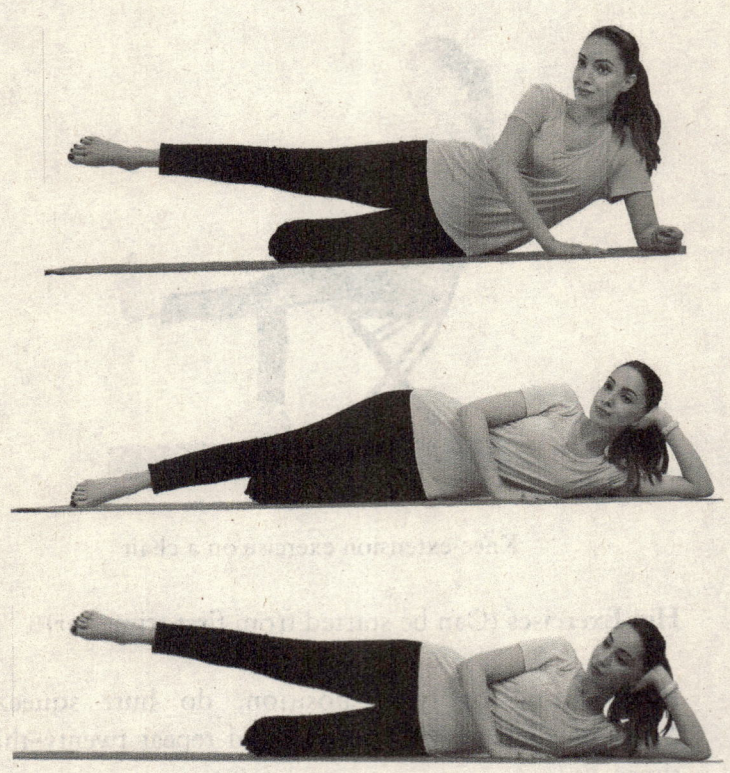

**Pelvic Tilts** (Can be started from the first trimester in a lying position)

Stand straight with the support of a ball or against a wall and perform pelvic tilts. Anterior tilting will counterbalance the already posterior tilted pelvis.

This can also be done by sitting on the edge of a chair at office or on the floor in a butterfly position.

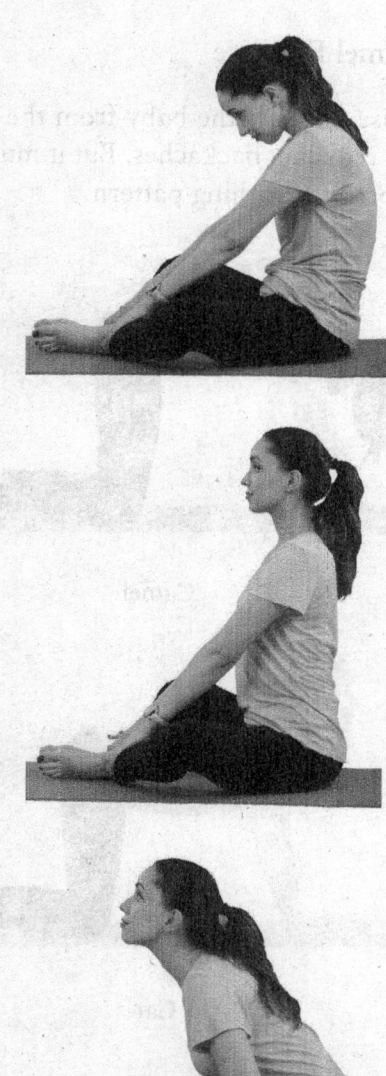

## Cat or Camel Exercise

This exercise offloads the baby from the spine. It is very effective in reducing backaches. But it must be performed with the correct breathing pattern.

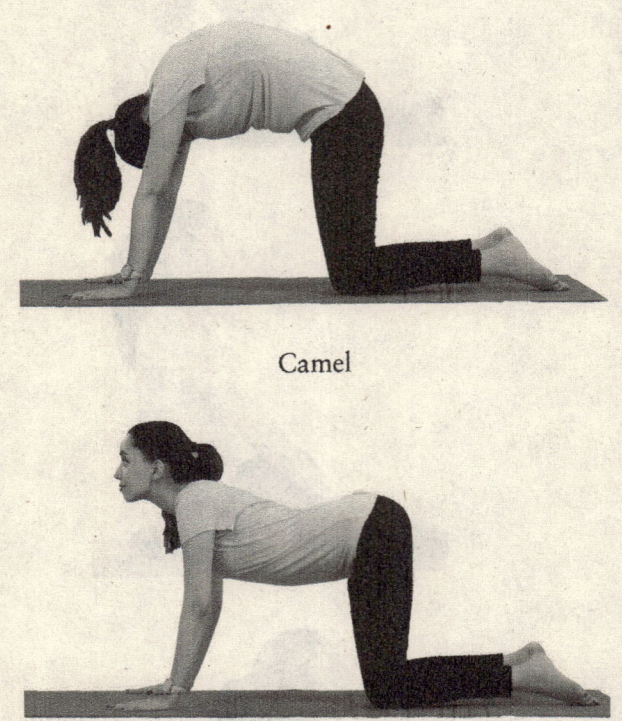

Camel

Cat

## Neck Exercises

Perform side-to-side neck movement and rotation. Repeat each ten times. Also, combine neck isometrics.

Keep your hand on your forehead and press your head against it while doing the same with your hand. Hold for five seconds and then relax. Repeat the same on the left side, right side and behind the head.

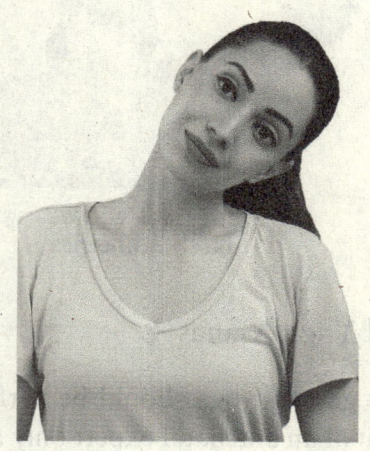

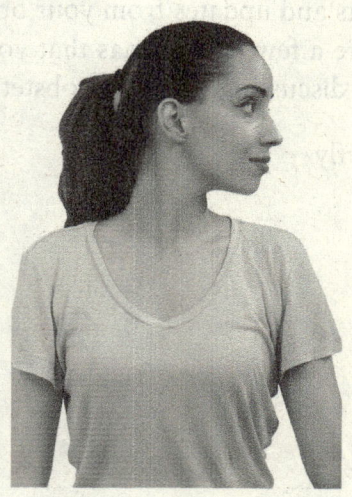

Neck bending and rotation

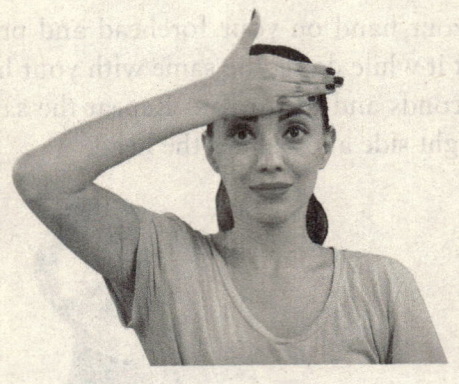

Neck isometrics

## Antenatal Yoga Asanas

Ideally, pregnancy yoga should be performed under the supervision of an antenatal expert only after analysing all your reports and updates from your obstetrician.

Here are a few easy asanas that you may perform at home after discussing with your obstetrician.

Half-Butterfly

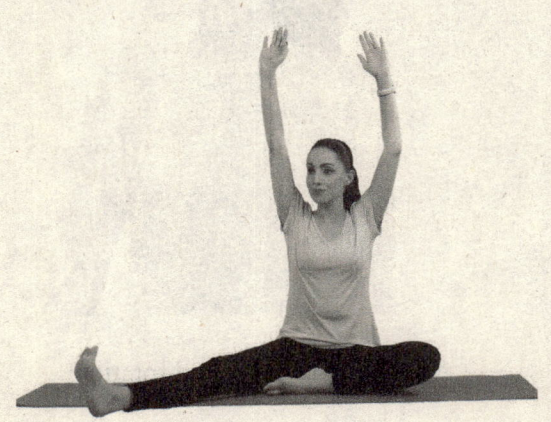

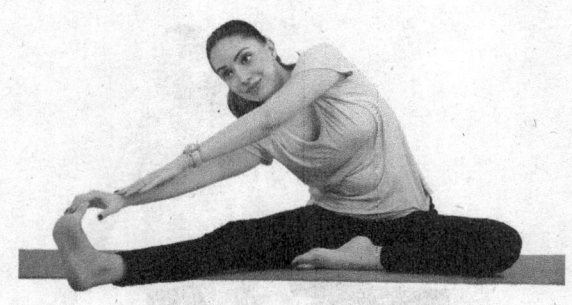

Bend sideways to avoid pressure on your bump

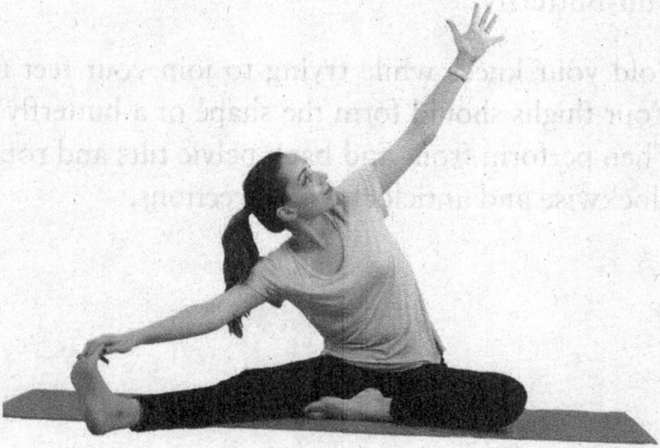

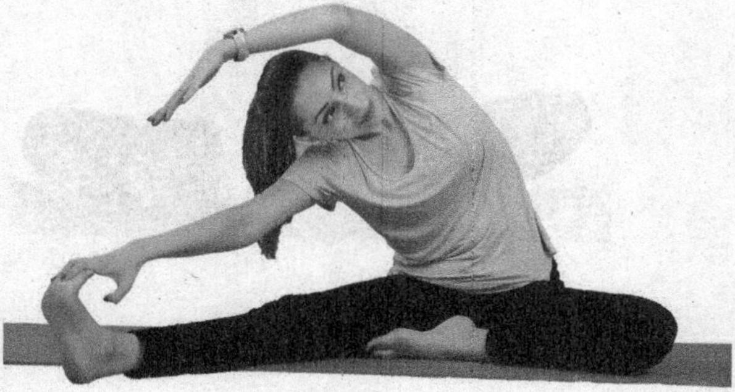

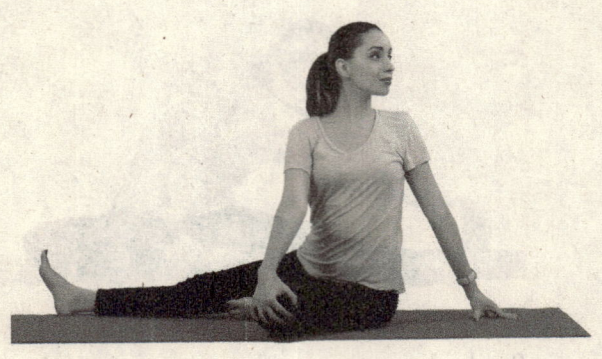

## Full-Butterfly

Fold your knees while trying to join your feet together. Your thighs should form the shape of a butterfly's wings. Then perform front and back pelvic tilts and rotations in clockwise and anticlockwise directions.

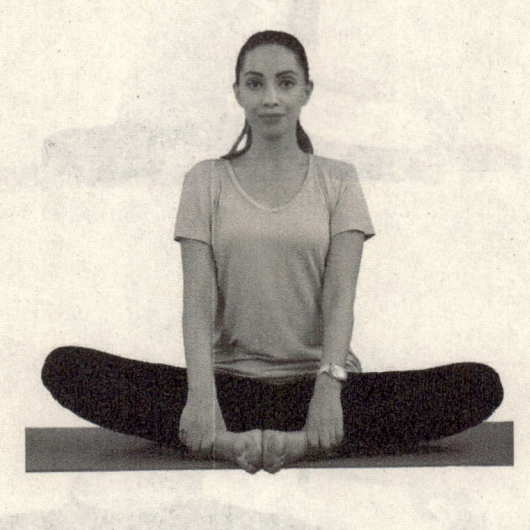

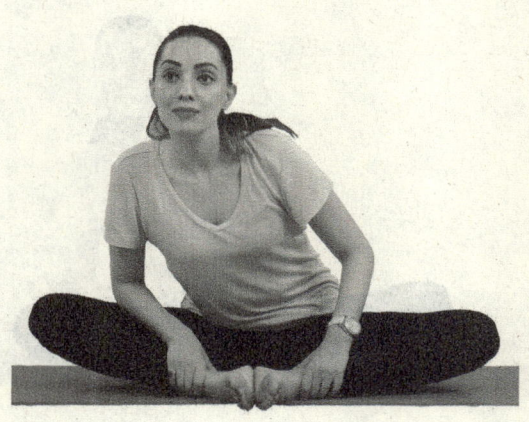

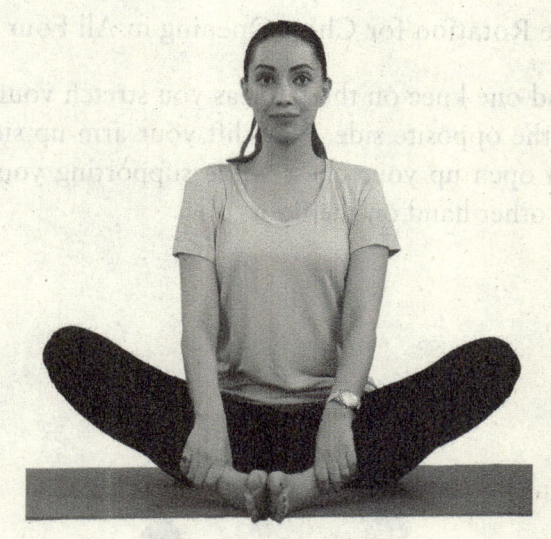

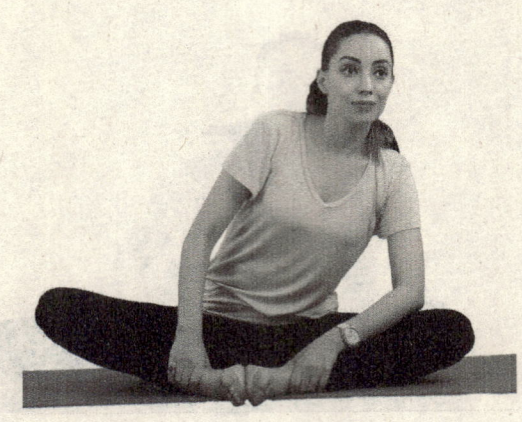

## Side Rotation for Chest Opening in All Four Positions

Bend one knee on the floor as you stretch your other leg on the opposite side. Now lift your arm up sideways as you open up your chest while supporting yourself with the other hand on the floor.

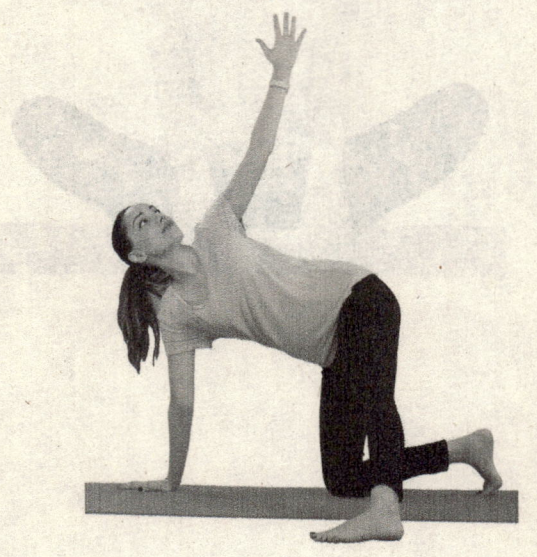

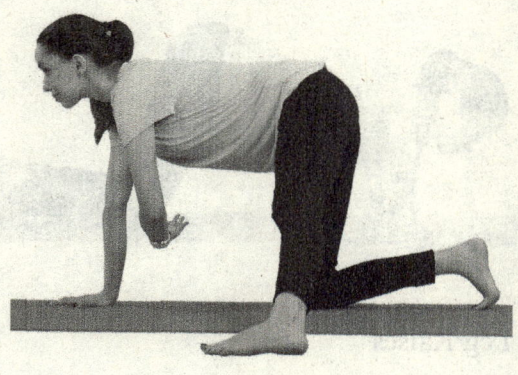

## Push-ups for Strengthening Chest and Upper Body

Place your knees on the floor as you stretch your arms, with your elbows bent at a ninety-degree angle, placing both your hands on the floor. Now move your upper body up and down.

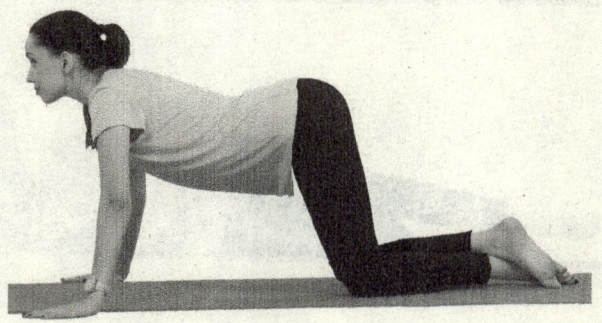

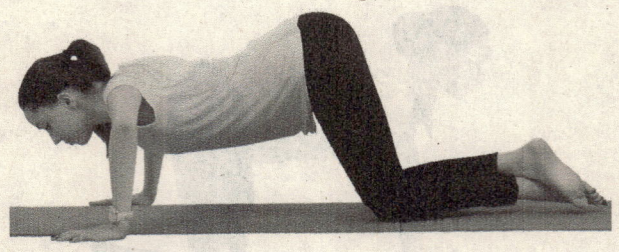

## Side Leg Raises

Lie down on your side with the support of one hand and lift your leg upwards. Don't try to lift it too high.

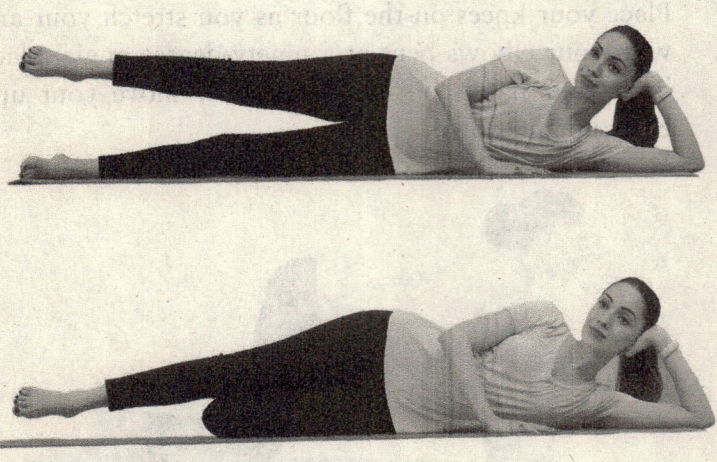

## Side Leg, Knee to Shoulder

As you lie down on your side, bend your knee upwards towards your shoulder.

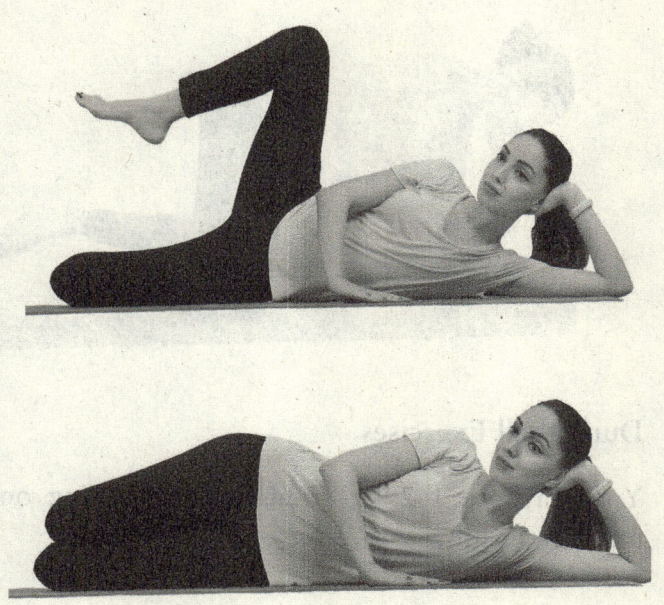

## Hip Rotation in All Four Positions

As you place yourself in all four positions with your hands supported on the floor and knees bent, lift one knee off the floor and rotate it clockwise.

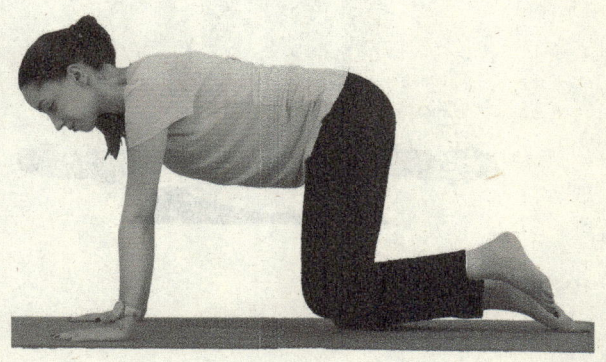

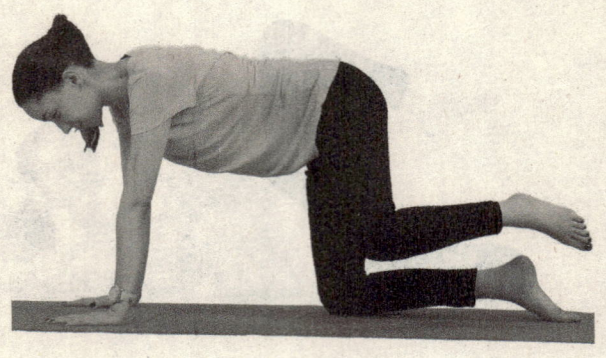

## Dumb-bell Exercises

You may use 1–2 kg dumb-bells depending on your muscle strength.

## Biceps Curl

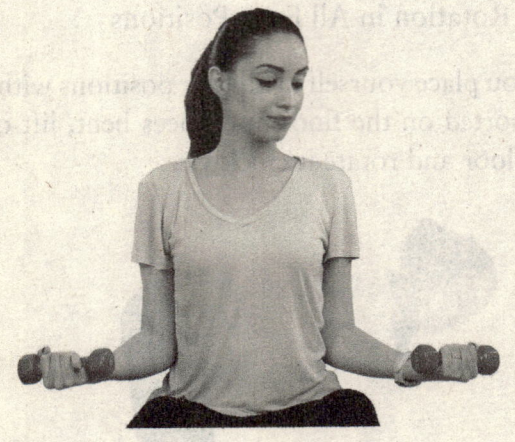

Triceps

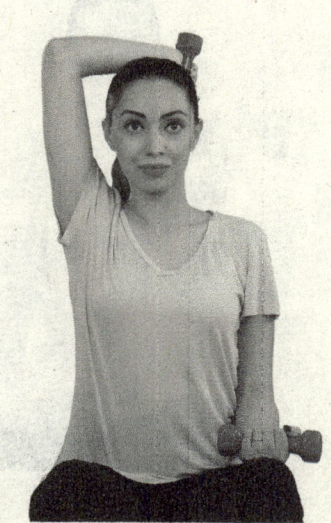

Shoulders

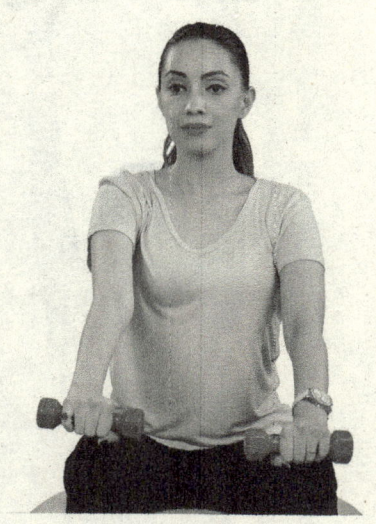

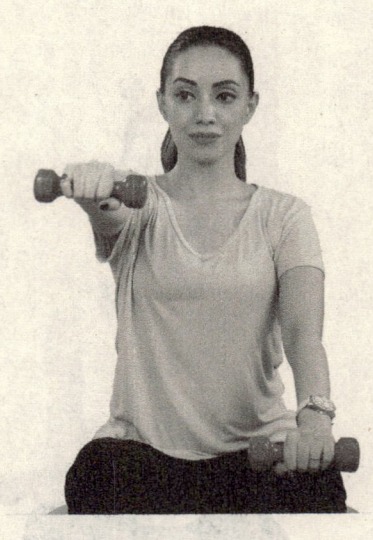

Overhead

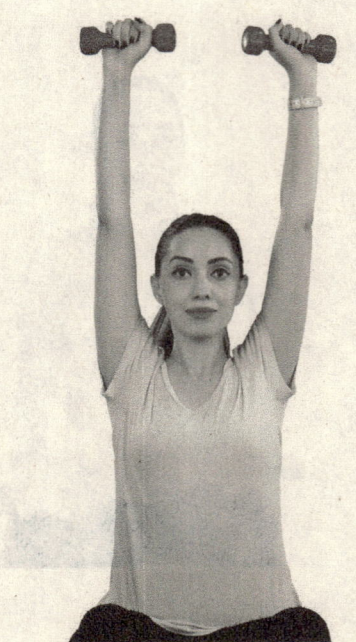

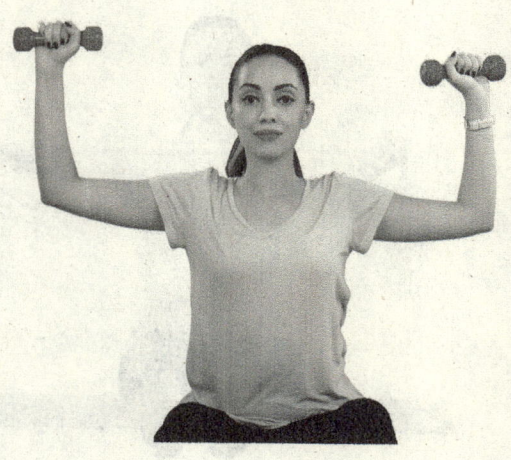

**Theraband Exercises** (Upper body exercises along with breathing)

Stretching and Releasing

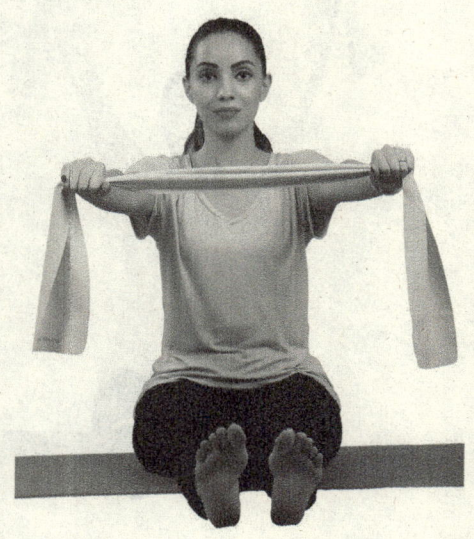

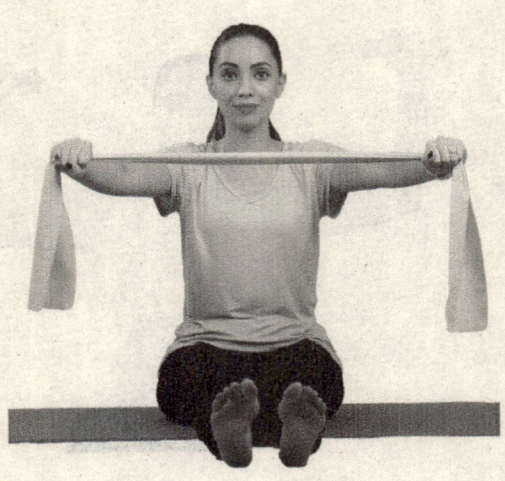

Pulling and Moving Arms up

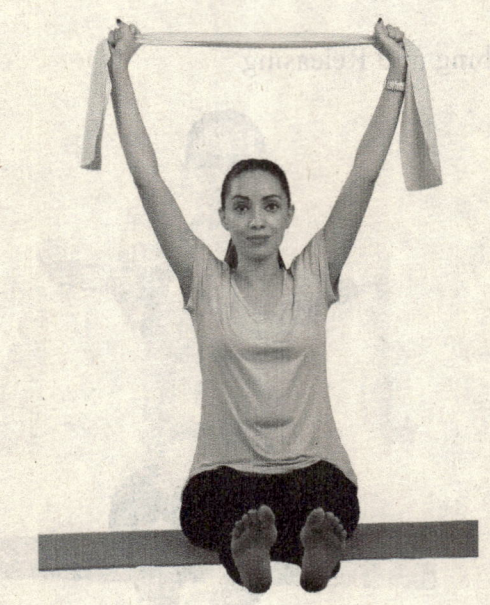

# Bow and Arrow

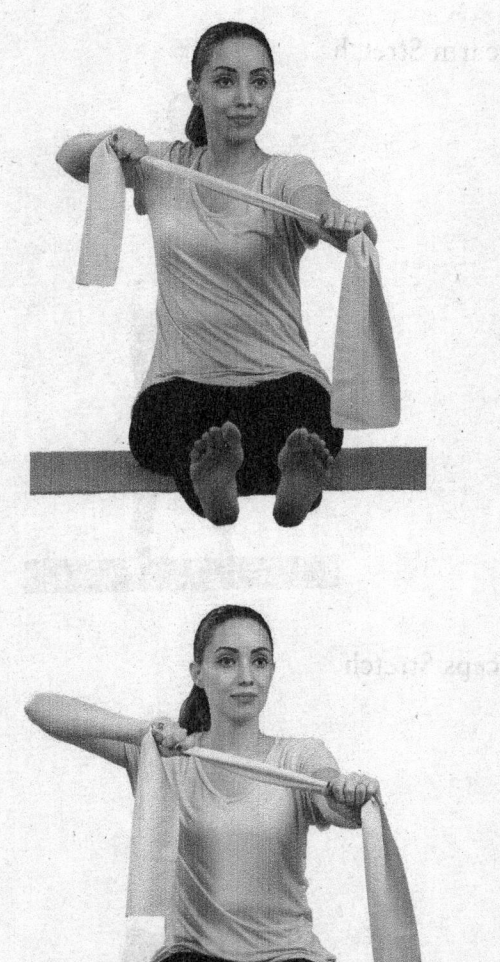

# Stretches

## Forearm Stretch

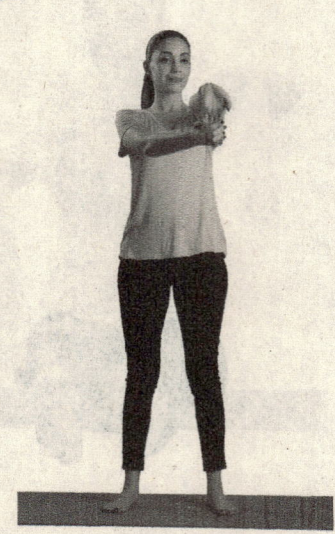

## Triceps Stretch

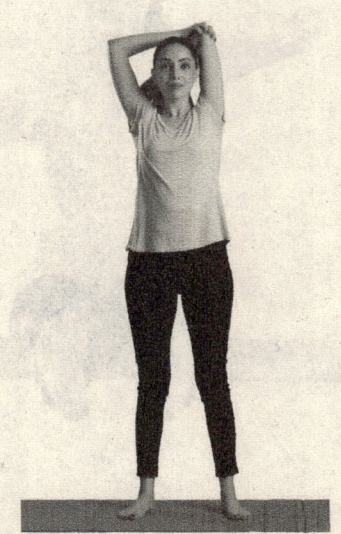

## Thigh Stretch

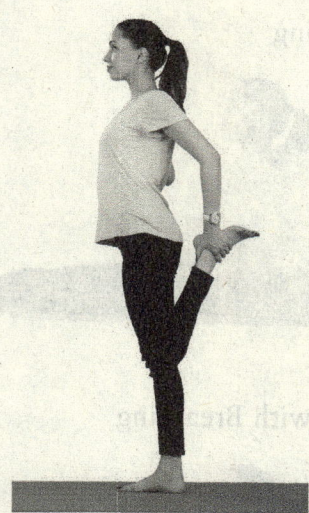

## Calf Stretch

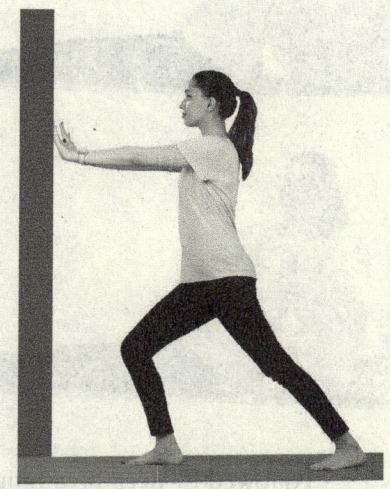

## Breathing with Swiss Ball

### Deep Breathing

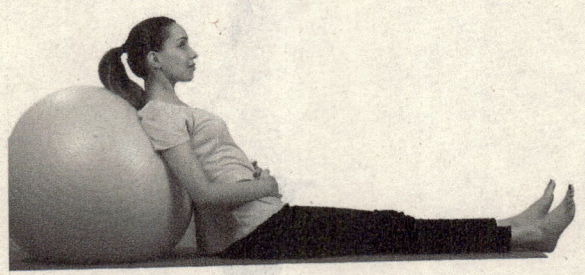

### Side-to-side with Breathing

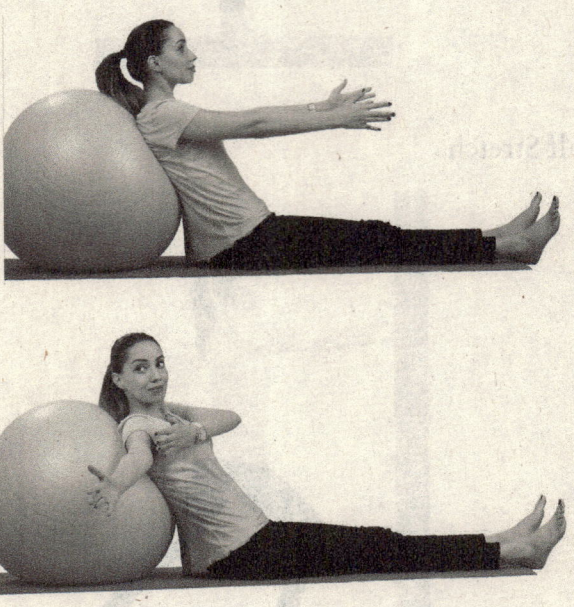

Followed by deep breathing

## Interlock Fingers behind Head

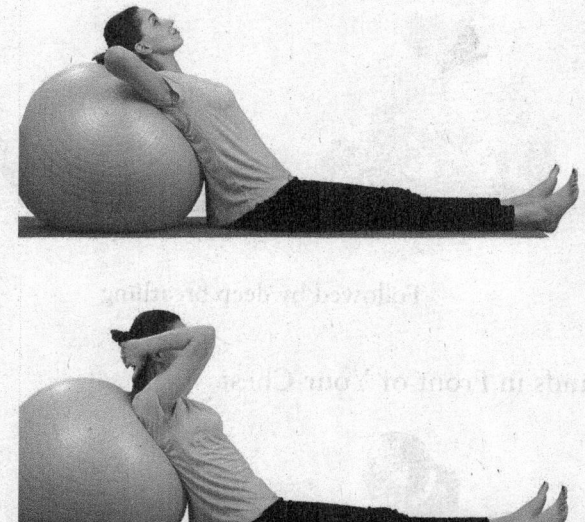

Followed by deep breathing

## Interlock Fingers, Stretch Arms up

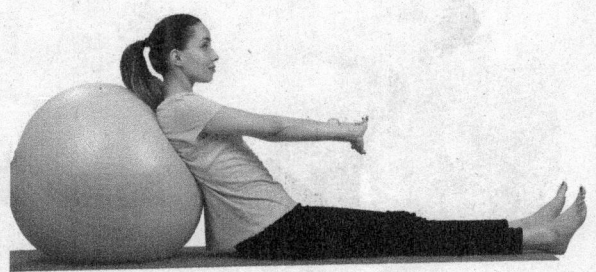

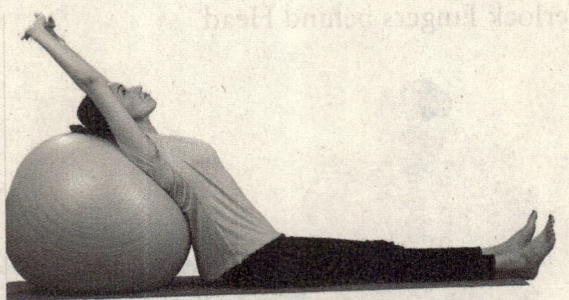

Followed by deep breathing

## Hands in Front of Your Chest

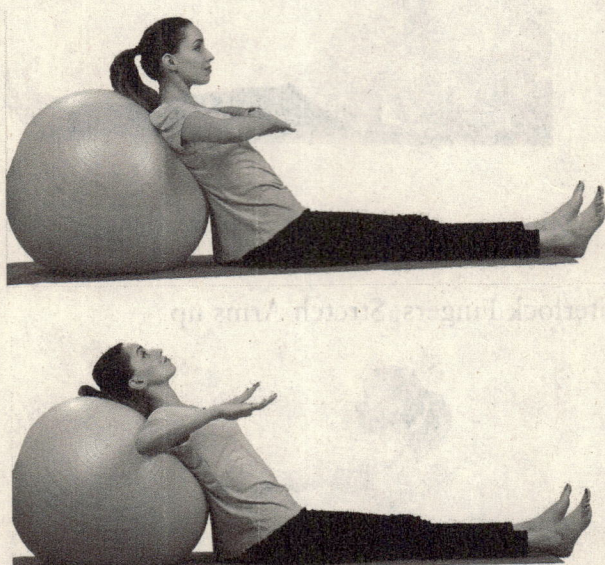

Followed by deep breathing

## Are You Sleeping Right?

A lot of patients walk into my OPD complaining of severe backaches while tossing in bed or after waking up in the morning. This could be due to the wrong sleeping position. Sleeping the right way during pregnancy is very important to prevent backaches and to maintain a good supply of blood flow to your baby.

Choose to lie sideways after five months or when your obstetrician tells you to do so. It is advisable to sleep on your left side as against lying on your back. Sleeping on your back will make the enlarged uterus press the vena cava, the vein that brings the blood back to the heart and can affect circulation in both the mother and to the baby. So it is better to use a three-pillow support system.

Pregnancy pillows are also available in the market and online. You may simply use a bolster under your upper leg to raise it, maintaining it at a ninety-degree angle at the hip and the knee. Let the lower leg be straight. Use a small cushion under the baby bump. This will also prevent too much stretching of the core muscles, hence reducing sagging of the belly. It will also avoid straining of the back. A regular pillow under the head and shoulders will keep the heart level raised, providing a steady circulation to the baby at night as she starts compressing the vena cava while growing.

Remember, sleeping right is very important to enjoy a healthy and fit pregnancy.

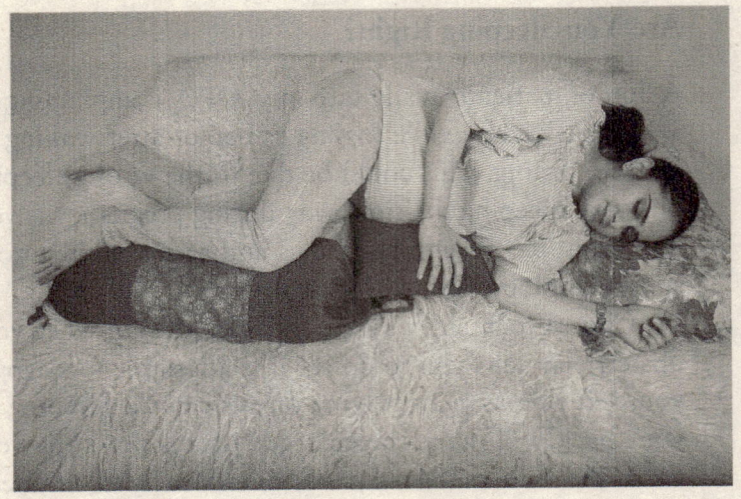

# 6

# Mood Swings

The very normal mood swings in pregnancy can take your emotions to places they have never been before—exhilarating highs and depressing lows. You can be over the moon one moment and down in the dumps the next, weeping inexplicably over insurance commercials. Can you blame it on your hormones? You bet! These swings maybe more pronounced in the first trimester (when hormonal havoc is at its peak) and, in general, in women who ordinarily suffer from marked emotional ups and downs before their periods (it's sort of like pre-menstrual syndrome but pumped up).

Conflicting feelings about a pregnancy once it's confirmed might make you even more temperamental. Marked physical changes during this time is also likely to overwhelm you.

Mood swings tend to moderate somewhat after the first trimester, once hormone levels calm down a little—and once you have adjusted to some of those changes (you will never adjust to all of them). In the meantime, though there's no sure way to hop off that emotional roller coaster, there are several ways to minimize the mood mayhem.

- **Keep Your Blood Sugar up:** What does blood sugar have to do with moods? A lot! Dips in blood sugar, caused by long gaps between meals, can lead to mood crashes. Yet another compelling reason to ditch your usual three meals a day and switch to six. But by sugar I obviously don't mean indulging in sweets.
- **Cut down on Sugar and Caffeine:** That candy bar, that doughnut, that bottle of Coca Cola will give your blood sugar a quick spike followed by a plunge that will take your mood along with it. Caffeine has the same effect, adding to mood instability. So limit both for happier results.
- **Eat Well:** In general, eating well will help you feel your best emotionally as well as physically. Follow your diet as best as you can. Get plenty of omega-3 fatty acids in your diet (walnuts, fish and enriched eggs, to name a few). They might help moderate your mood; they are also important for your baby's brain development.
- **Move around Frequently:** The more you move, the better will be your mood. That's because exercise releases feel-good endorphins that can send your spirits soaring. Consult your ob–gyn if you can start exercising.
- **Make Love:** If you are in the mood for love (and when not busy puking), making love can turn that frown

upside down. Sex releases happy hormones. It will also bring you closer to your partner at a time when your relationship could be facing new challenges. If sex isn't on the cards, cuddling, pillow talk and holding hands can also boost your mood.

- **Light up Your Life:** Research has shown that sunlight can actually lighten moods. Sun yourself regularly (just don't forget to apply a sunscreen first).
- **Talk about It:** Worried? Anxious? Feeling unsettled? Talk about your feelings to your partner (who's probably feeling plenty of the same things), to friends, to other pregnant women on online pregnancy message boards. You might end up feeling normal after all.
- **Rest:** Fatigue can exacerbate the mood swings. Make sure you are getting enough sleep (but not too much, since that can make you feel more fatigued and emotionally unstable). Learn to relax. Stress can definitely take your moods down, so find ways of moderating it.

If there is one person in your life who's more affected and bewildered by your mood swings than you, it is your partner. Once your partner understands why you are acting the way you are, they might be able to help you better. Tell them what you need (more help around the house? A night out at your favourite restaurant?) and what you don't need (comments on your posterior, picking up after him), what makes you feel better and what makes you feel worse. And be specific. Even the most loving partner can't read your mind.

Just remember that mood swings in pregnancy are normal. Prepare your partner for them. Let them know you might shout or cry without any visible reason. They shouldn't fan the flames and just let the storm blow away.

# 7

# Relaxation Techniques

It's common to feel anxious thinking about childbirth and the changes in your life after it. But you need to relax and there are exercises that can help you soothe your nerves. Practise them for 10–15 minutes twice a day for optimum results.

Doing these exercises after waking up will help you stay happy and positive throughout the day. Performing these exercises at bedtime will ensure that you get a good sleep. This is especially important during the second trimester when a lot of women have difficulty falling asleep. Relaxation exercises are particularly beneficial to working women as it alleviates stress.

Close your eyes and think of something that makes you feel good and continue thinking about it. Inhale a lungful of air and then relax your jaws as you exhale. There is an interesting connection between your jaws and your vagina. The more relaxed your jaws the more will your vaginal muscles relax. A resting body prevents tightness of muscles. Remember, you will be able to deliver more easily if you are relaxed than if you are stiff.

Here are some techniques that you can practise to relax your body:

## Breathing with Full Body Relaxation or Deep Breathing

Relax your body and let your eyes close on their own. Inhale deeply while sticking out your abdomen and exhale as if you are blowing off a candle; your abdomen should go in. To feel the abdomen movements better and to know if you are doing them right, place your hands on your tummy as if you are hugging your baby and focus on the actions. Perform this for at least ten–fifteen times in a go.

## Rainbow Technique

In a sitting or a lying position, keep your eyes closed and picture the colours of a rainbow—violet, indigo, blue, green, yellow, orange and red.

Imagine yourself in a pool of red roses, feeling their softness and fragrance, and let your body float in it, relaxing your face, shoulders, chest, abdomen, hips, thighs and feet.

Imagine yourself in a pool of orange slush and feel it flowing over your face, chest, abdomen, hips, thighs and feet. Think about your baby trying to drink some too. Well, it is vitamin C so we don't mind either.

Or you could picture sunning yourself on a beach. Feel the warmth on your face, neck, shoulders, arms, chest, abdomen, legs and feet. Your baby is enjoying the sun as well. As it is vitamin D, we definitely want the baby to get some too.

Another lovely image to conjure up is picturing yourself on a bed of damp grass.

Or you could imagine yourself on a boat on the sea. Enjoy the blue sky and the waves. Inhale deeply and relax your body.

## Alphabet Technique

Now it's time for some visual learning. As you inhale, picture entering an imaginary field from the left side in a wave-like motion with a capital letter of the English alphabet followed by the lower case one behind. As you exhale, picture the letters leaving from the right side. Imagine the twenty-six letters gradually. You can also do this with your partner. Ask them to randomly tell you any letter and picture it accordingly.

## Counting Technique

Start counting as you inhale; reverse count when you exhale. All these techniques can be combined with music therapy and practised especially at bedtime or early in the morning for better results.

## Facial Relaxation

Achieving deep facial relaxation is very important as it sets the tone for the rest of your body.

Lie on the bed and close your eyes gradually. Try to be aware of the muscles in and around your eyes. Your eyelids should droop naturally. This is when you'll sense relaxation spreading down from your forehead to your eyes, cheekbones and finally around your jaws. Let your lower jaw recede as your teeth part. Your eyelids will feel heavier as your cheeks and jaws go limp. Place the tip of your tongue at your palate; try to connect with the energy orbit in your body. Feel your head making a dent in the pillow. As you practise this technique, you will feel your neck, shoulders and elbows drooping. Picture your shoulders opening outwards and sinking into the frame of your body as you relax further.

Prepare for relaxation in labour by ensuring that you practise ten minutes of relaxation daily.

# 8

# Gestational Diabetes

Gestational diabetes is an important concern during pregnancy. It can mostly show up around the middle of the second trimester or even later. If required, your ob–gyn may suggest that you get tested for it. As the symptoms of gestational diabetes aren't prominent, your healthcare provider may offer a screening test between the twenty-fourth and twenty-eighth week of your pregnancy. If you have any risk factors for the disease, your provider may suggest doing the test earlier.

The most common test is the oral glucose screening test. It measures the efficiency with which your body produces insulin. On the day of the test, your healthcare provider will give you a sweet liquid to drink. An hour later, a blood test will be done to check your glucose levels.

If the results indicate high blood sugar, you'll have to take a longer test called the oral glucose tolerance test. For this one, you'll have to fast overnight after which you will again be given a sweet liquid to drink. Your blood will be tested at fasting, then again after 1–3 hours. If the results of both the tests show that your blood sugar is too high, you'll be diagnosed with gestational diabetes.

Sugar enters the baby through the placenta. Gestational diabetes may lead to the formation of more insulin in the pancreas of the baby. After birth, the baby can run the risk of developing hypoglycaemia. Uncontrolled gestational diabetes might also lead to the baby being overweight at the time of birth. Also, not only is the growth of the baby affected, the disease also raises the risk of having a premature birth.

If you are suffering from gestational diabetes, you will need to pay extra attention to your health to ensure that the sugar levels remain under control. Your ob–gyn will keep a check on the baby's growth during antenatal visits and through ultrasound scans and other tests, if required.

Exercising and a healthy diet are particularly helpful in controlling sugar levels. As and when you're allowed to exercise make sure that you are regular, and eat healthy.

Prenatal yoga, breathing exercises and walking are all very beneficial at this time. You might feel lazy sometimes but you must make sure to exercise at least three–four times a week.

## 9

# Supplements in Pregnancy

Getting enough nourishment is a non-negotiable priority during pregnancy. The formation and development of the baby hinges on this. But sometimes homemade food fails to meet our daily quota of nutrition. Deficiencies are on the rise these days as our food is no longer as fresh off the earth as it was fifty years ago, thanks to modernization. Nutritional supplements help bolster our system by supplying the missing nourishment. Some of the important ones that you should take are listed below.

## Folic Acid

Even before conception, your ob–gyn might prescribe some folic acid supplements if required. Folic acid helps in preventing neural tube defects and any serious abnormalities of the brain and spinal cord. The risk of developing these abnormalities usually increases with the age at which you conceive. So if you are above thirty, you might be asked to take folic acid supplements. But there are natural sources for deriving this as well, such as leafy green vegetables, beans, peas, milk or eggs.

## Iron

Your blood volume will increase during pregnancy as the baby needs more blood supply for her body as well. There needs to be a corresponding increase of iron in your blood. Iron deficiency can make you feel fatigued and tired. So your ob–gyn might put you on iron supplements. Do not skip them. If you start experiencing diarrhoea or constipation after taking the supplements, discuss it with your ob–gyn. She will change the supplement; don't discontinue on your own. The natural sources for deriving iron are chicken, fish, eggs, beans, peas, lentils, carrots, beetroots, pomegranates, apples and dates.

## Protein

Proteins are crucial for the growth of your baby, especially during the second and third trimesters. But many women who eat plant-based food don't get substantial proteins during pregnancy. In this case, you might be put on a protein powder supplement. You must take it. Again, do not discontinue on your own; if you don't like the taste, there are lots of options available in the market. But do discuss it with your healthcare provider first. In addition to supplements, you should increase your intake of daal, eggs, milk, peas, curd, paneer, chicken, fish, etc., as these are natural sources of various proteins.

## Calcium

Calcium is a must for strong bones and teeth. If there isn't enough calcium, the baby will start taking it from your bones, which could lead to the development of osteoporosis in your life. So make sure you have a good amount of calcium in your diet. Try to drink about two–three glasses of milk daily, along with other milk-based products such as curd, paneer or lassi.

If you are a non-dairy person, inform your ob–gyn about it. She may put you on some calcium supplements if required.

## Vitamin D

Vitamin D deficiency is very common and found in people irrespective of their gender and age. You might be put on supplements if it is found that you do not get enough of this vitamin. A natural source of vitamin D is sunlight, so be sure to sun yourself adequately. As it is a fat-soluble vitamin, you need a good amount of healthy fat in your diet to absorb it despite the supplements. For a pregnant woman, about one teaspoon of ghee every day is good if there are no cardiac problems or cholesterol issues, which are anyway rare among pregnant women.

Do not combine iron and calcium supplements together. Calcium reduces the absorption of iron. Take your iron supplements along with a glass of lemon water as vitamin C enhances the absorption of iron. Do not take it with milk. You can take your calcium supplement with milk in the morning.

# 10

# What to Avoid?

## Caffeine

Too much caffeine is not good for the baby, so its intake must be checked. Caffeine in the form of chocolates, coffee, coke, tea or other food items is daily consumed by us. During pregnancy, you should cut down on it. It's safe to consume around two cups of tea or a cup of coffee in a day, along with a small slab of chocolate if you crave for it. Even if you work at night and in order to keep yourself awake, take coffee throughout the day, you need to watch every cup that you pick up. Avoid aerated drinks.

## Green Tea

We know that green tea is very good for health. But how safe it is for the baby, we are not really sure. I personally play safe and advise my patients not to have green tea during pregnancy. If you must, have one cup a day. You could switch to Chamomile tea instead, which is proven to provide excellent results in pregnancy. I advise my patients to have a cup of Chamomile tea daily, especially in the evenings during the third trimester.

## Alcohol

Many patients ask me if they can have just one glass of wine during pregnancy. Why take unnecessary risks? I advise them to not have any alcohol during this time. In fact, avoid alcohol for as long as you are breastfeeding. You must restrict yourself; avoid going to places where alcohol is easily accessible. Take your partner's help in this.

## Smoking

Smoking can have extremely harmful effects on the baby. In fact, I tell my patients to even avoid passive smoking. Make it a rule to keep your home smoke-free. If your partner or anyone at home smokes, tell them that maybe it's time for them to switch to a healthy habit.

## Medications

Self-medication is dangerous during pregnancy and puts you at an increased risk of miscarriage. Please do not take any medicine without consulting your ob–gyn or physician. Do not take any over-the-counter medicine without consulting your healthcare provider.

# 11

# Learning Time for
# Your Baby in the Womb

It is important to do activities that build your baby's learning and developmental skills. As she grows inside the womb, she will start responding to the external environment towards the third trimester onwards—she will respond to light, sound, touch and can start experiencing emotions like happiness, sadness, excitement and so on. Your baby can be playful at time, giving you constant kicks, and not move at all sometimes.

Babies can be very moody even inside the womb. A classic example is when you visit your radiologist for an ultrasound and hear her say: 'I am unable to see the baby completely as she is not ready to move or change her position.' External environments have an effect on the mood of the baby. Here are some activities to enhance the sensory stimulation of the baby inside the womb.

## How Colour Benefits You and Your Baby during Pregnancy and Birth

Colour therapy has been proven to be beneficial in various treatment plans. Imagine if everything around us was just in shades of black. What impact would it have on us? We need light to enjoy colours around us. Nice bright colours can elevate our mood while the dull ones can keep us cold at heart. Now do you understand why playschools' classrooms are so vibrant and colourful? Babies get bored pretty fast. Exposing them to different bright colours keeps them excited, happy and joyful.

### Introducing Colours to Your Baby

- Try to play with lots of colours. Use crayons and make some paintings. It's an excellent way to ensure relaxation of your mind as well. It helps in reducing your anxieties and fears about childbirth, if any.
- Towards the end of your second trimester, you may even enrol for art classes once or twice a week.

### Wearing Colours

- Wear colourful clothes.
- Choose a different colour each day.
- The whole week can be divided into the seven rainbow colours.
- Stay bright and chirpy during pregnancy.

The colours you choose to wear can also affect your mood—bright colours keep mood swings away.

## Eating Colourful Food

- Add a lot of colourful items to your bowl of salad and fruits.
- Add yellow, green or red pepper, broccoli, corn, cherry tomatoes, cucumbers, zucchini, lettuce, kiwi, oranges, lemon and apples to your daily bowl of antioxidants.

However, do not get too carried away and drink colourful, aerated drinks as they contain a high level of sugar.

## Cooking

Cooking can be very recreational for women who don't do it regularly. A more exciting idea would be to join a cookery or a baking class.

## Reading

My favourite recreational activity is reading. Avoid e-books as you don't want unwanted strain on your eyes during pregnancy. If you are a working woman, try taking out time to read on weekends. If you are a homemaker, try to read daily. Make it a routine. The best thing to do is to read at bedtime. It will also help you fall asleep. Among others, you can read:

## Pregnancy Books

Congratulations, as you are already reading one. Read as you gain lots of useful information. ☺

## Parenting Books

I advise my patients to read at least one book on parenting during pregnancy. It might be helpful to read a book on the early phase of a newborn to understand what is normal and what isn't. For a new mother, there are so many facts that you need to know. Educate yourself now as there isn't going to be any time once your baby arrives, trust me!

## Baby Storybooks

Read out stories to your baby in your third trimester and feel her responding with some movements.

# Listen to Music

There are many tracks available online for pregnant women. Listen to such pieces daily. Try to continue this habit even after delivery. You should listen to nursery rhymes in your third trimester. Your baby will respond to these by kicking. Download the rhymes or buy some CDs. These can be used later as your child is growing up. At home, you should play these on speakers instead of listening through headphones. You can listen to them while driving and at lunch breaks at work too.

## Play Games and Solve Puzzles

We already know that puzzles are fantastic brain exercisers. You should solve puzzles or play Sudoku to enhance your brain and your baby's too.☺ Play games daily; solve crossword or other activities. Start at the beginner's level if you find the advanced ones daunting.

Playing snakes and ladder, ludo, monopoly, scrabble and other board games are fun and effective exercises. You could play any safe indoor games as well. Pregnancy is no sickness, remember. Try to cherish it as much as possible.

# 12

# The Third Trimester

As your due date nears, you will get anxious and have frequent mood swings. So make an effort to keep yourself happy despite the change in your body shape and the numerous visits to the washroom. By this stage, your body should be used to the changes. Some more are in the offing.

## Braxton Hicks Contractions

These are contractions that appear as a slight tightness around your abdomen. They tend to get stronger and more frequent as your reach your nine month.

Tip—Do breathing exercises whenever you feel them.

## Aches and Pains

Due to weight gain and changes in your spinal curve, you might experience a mild pain in your back and legs.

Tip—Lots of regular exercises like prenatal yoga, stretches, ball exercises and theraband exercises are helpful.

## Shortness of Breath

You might easily get breathless while talking for too long or climbing stairs at work.

Tip—Practise lots of deep breathing and stamina-building exercises.

## Acidity/Heartburn

As your uterus rises in the initial part of the third trimester, you might experience heartburn in the evenings. It gradually gets better as the uterus starts descending while preparing to position the baby in the pelvis for labour towards the thirty-fifth week.

Tip—Take Chamomile tea and light meals after 4 p.m. Do light walking after your meals to aid digestion.

## Excessive Urination

As your baby puts pressure on your bladder, you will make frequent visits to the loo from the thirty-second week onwards. It might get super annoying to pee almost every other hour but don't worry, it will be fine once the bladder gets relieved from the baby's weight after you deliver.

Tip—Do lots of Kegels.

## Some More Emotional Changes

Mixed feelings: The thought of childbirth at this stage can cause stress.

Tip—Prepare for childbirth. Refer to the chapters later that will guide you on labour.

Excitement: The thought of having your baby soon in your arms will get you excited. You will get an urge to keep everything clean for the arrival of your baby.

Tip—Stay calm and wait. ☺

## Varicose Veins

You are vulnerable to developing varicose veins if it runs in your family. They often seem to appear for the first time during pregnancy, and worsen in future pregnancies. This could be due to the increased blood volume that puts extra pressure on the blood vessels. The veins in your legs are especially affected as they have to work against gravity to push all that extra blood back up to your heart. Also, the growing uterus puts more pressure on your pelvic blood vessels.

The symptoms of varicose veins aren't that difficult to recognize but they vary in severity. You might experience mild or severe pain in your legs; heaviness in your legs or feet; some visible swelling that makes it difficult to wear closed footwear. You could develop some blue or purple colour patches on your legs and thighs as well. In severe cases, the skin above the veins becomes swollen, dry and irritated. Occasionally, superficial thrombophlebitis (or inflammation of a surface vein due to a blood clot) may develop at the site of varicosity, so always check with your ob–gyn about varicose veins symptoms.

Here are some precautions that you can take:

- Do not sit or stand for too long. Keep the blood flowing. When sitting, avoid crossing your legs and elevate them if possible. When lying down, raise your legs by placing a pillow under your feet. When resting or sleeping, try to lie on your left side, which is the best one for optimum circulation.

- Do not gain too much weight. Excess weight increases the demands on your already overworked circulatory system. Try to stay within the recommended guidelines.

- Do not lift heavy weights as they can make the affected veins bulge.

- Push gently during bowel movements. Putting too much pressure can cause a strain on those veins.

- Avoid wearing very tight clothes as they restrict your blood circulation and make it even more difficult for the blood to flow back upwards. Prefer flats over high heels.

- Get some exercise, such as a brisk 20–30 minute walk or yoga every day.

- Be sure that your diet includes plenty of foods rich in vitamin C, which helps keep your blood vessels healthy and elastic.

## Therapies to Help You during Your Third Trimester

The wait to receive your baby in your arms will keep you on your toes. Here are some great distraction tips that you can enjoy during your third trimester:

### Shopping Therapy

Indulge in some maternity shopping or buy for your baby shower; get skincare products to fight those skin and hair changes. Purchase children's books and make your partner read out nursery rhymes aloud to your baby at night.

### Salon or Spa Therapy

Give your skin some rejuvenation; pamper yourself with some nice aroma oils. Skin and hair care are important. You may have pregnancy-induced hair fall or skin pigmentation. So a light facial and head massage can be beneficial. Remember, no lying down on your back. Instead, opt for a chair or a pregnancy table. You might enjoy a light manicure or pedicure. Bending and cleaning your feet with a big bump is difficult so you might need some help. In case of a pedicure or foot massage, no reflexology points should be pressed in the sole. Only light touches are advisable till the thirty-sixth week.

## Music Therapy

Relaxing music, the chirping of birds, the flowing of water, the sound of wind blowing, or slow music should be played in your room or in your car. Maintain a slow, deep breathing pattern while listening to it. I strongly advise my patients to avoid playing loud and fast music after the thirty-second week.

## Diet in Third Trimester

It's important to have healthy food during this phase as your body starts preparing to breastfeed.

Early morning—One glass milk and nuts.

Breakfast—A boiled egg or sprouts; paneer sandwich.

Mid-morning—Fruits.

Noon—Coconut water.

Lunch—One–two rotis or a bowl of rice, daal, subzi, salad and curd.

Evening—A cup of Chamomile tea.

Late evening—A glass of milk with flax seeds or lassi, buttermilk.

Dinner—Soup and salad; a roti or brown rice with daal or chicken or paneer.

Bedtime—Milk and dates.

## Exercises in Third Trimester

Of course, exercising now becomes even more important as this is the last trimester and you need to prepare for labour. You have to add some stamina-building exercises now as you might experience breathlessness at this stage. Also, in case you have been on bed rest during the second trimester, check with your ob–gyn if you should start exercising now.

You should walk regularly for around thirty minutes as permitted by your obstetrician. I make my patients do weight training from the thirtieth week onwards with 2 kg dumb-bells for an upper body workout. It helps in improving endurance and toning the body. Also, this is the time you need to prepare your upper body for carrying the weight of your baby in your arms and for feeding after delivery. Many patients who skip this come to me with cervical neck pain and shoulder pain postnatally. Upper body workouts are important to prevent these kinds of pain after delivery.

I advise all the exercises that have been mentioned for the second trimester plus the following ones:

## Squatting and Lunges (If the baby is not breech)

Stand straight with your feet wide apart at a forty-five-degree angle. Now bend your knees ninety degrees but don't cross your ankles. Ball support makes it easier and uses the right thigh muscles to make your legs stronger.

Full squats can be done by completely bending your knees and going down.

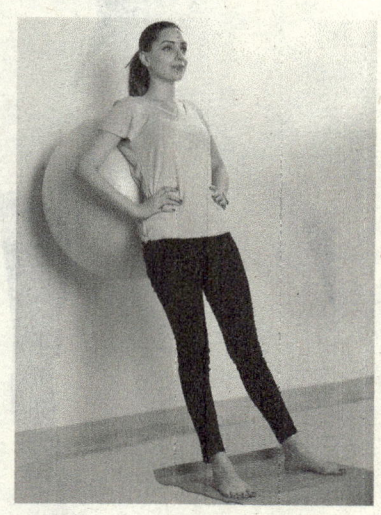

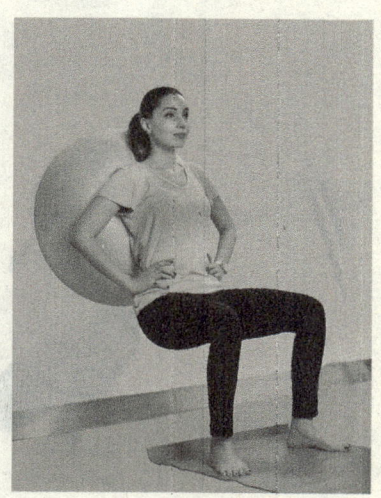

Squatting

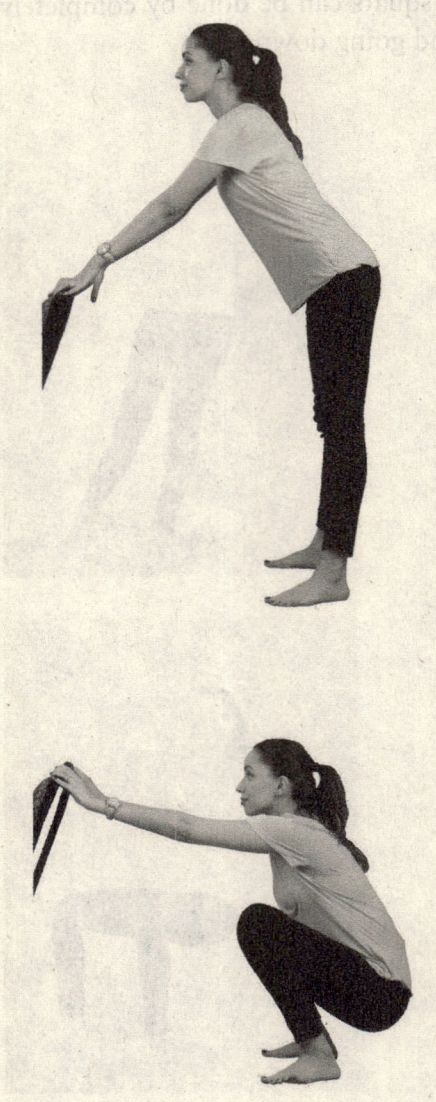

Lunges

## Lunges on Chair

Place one leg on a chair and bend your knee sideways.

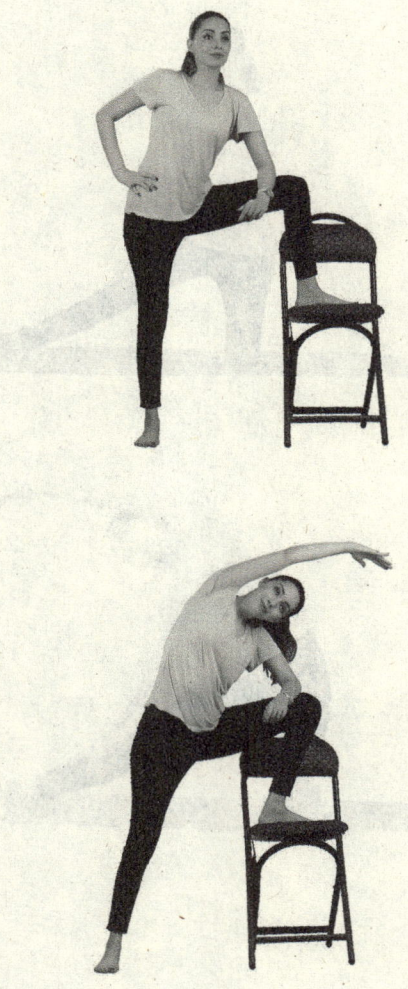

## Adductor Stretch with Wall Support on Floor

Place your leg against a wall and bend sideways in a kneeling position.

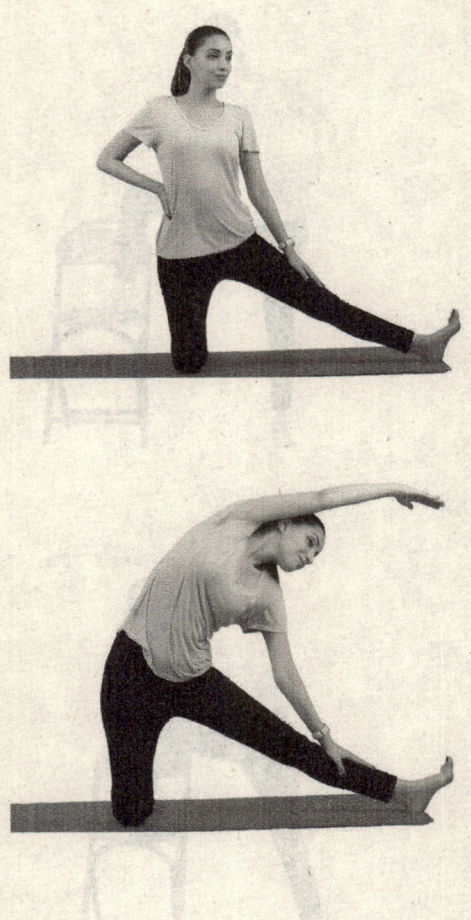

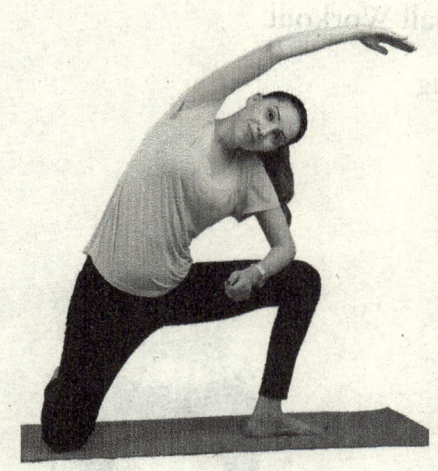

Back Stretch with a Chair, Legs Wide

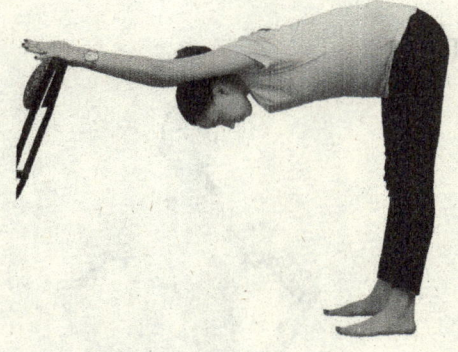

# Swiss Ball Workout

## Bouncing

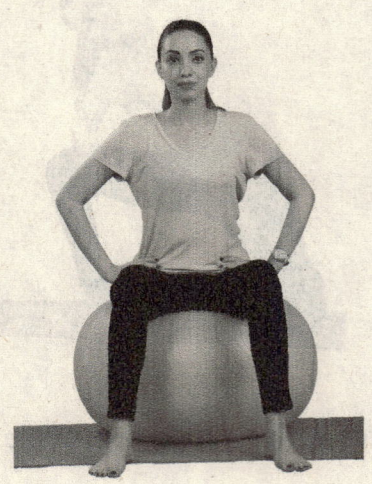

## Pelvic Tilts

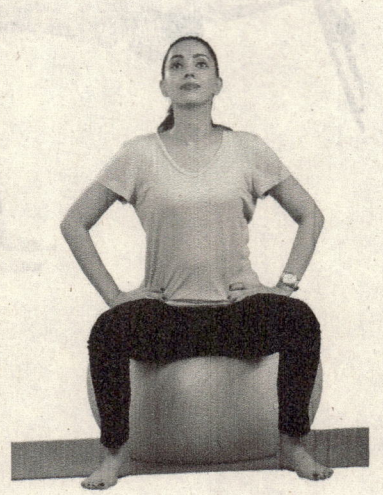

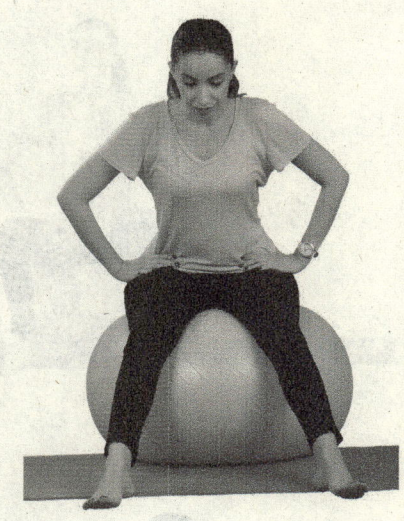

Side-to-side

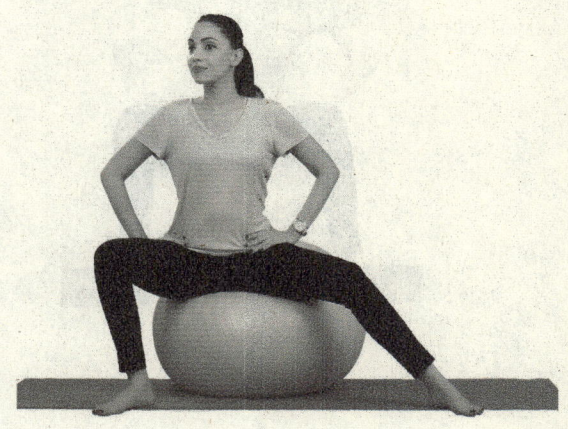

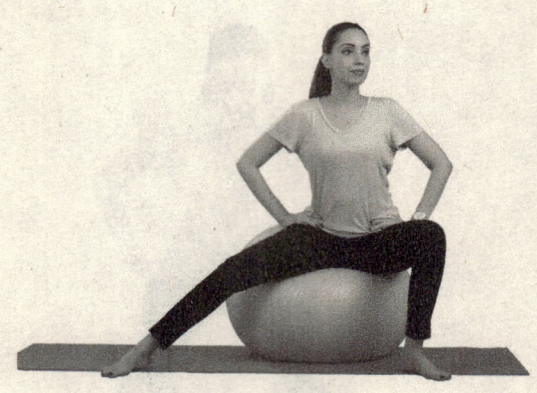

Rotation

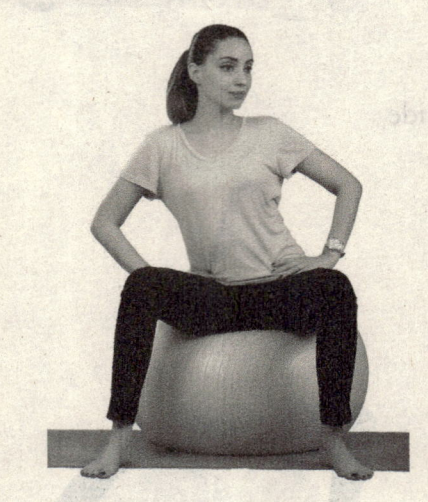

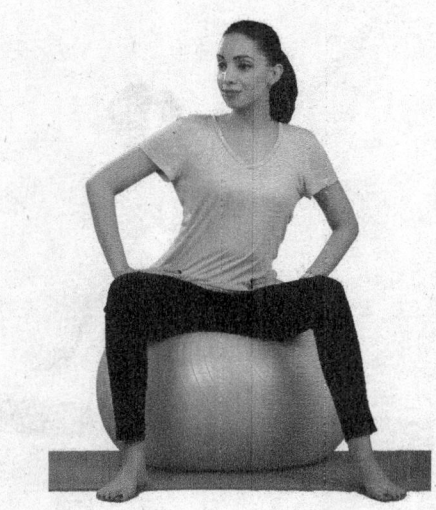

## Side Bends

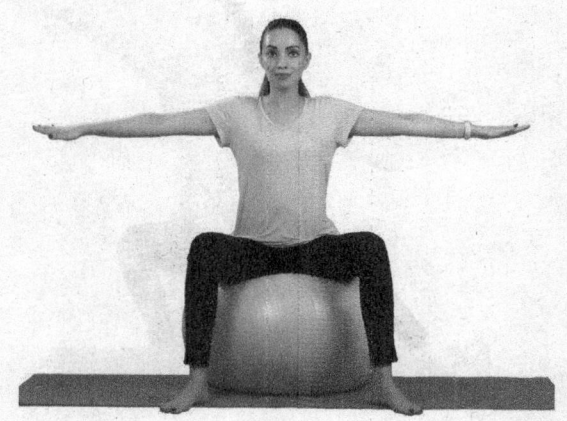

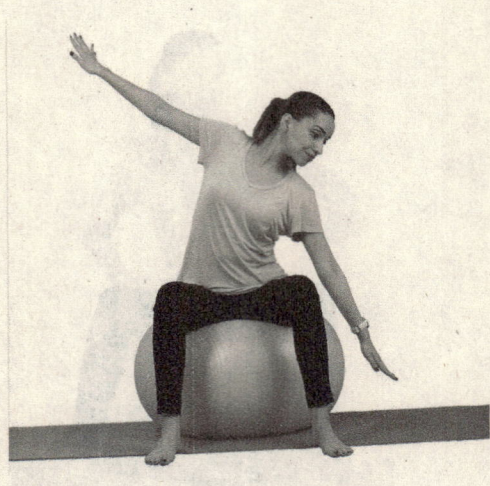

Arms Reach out

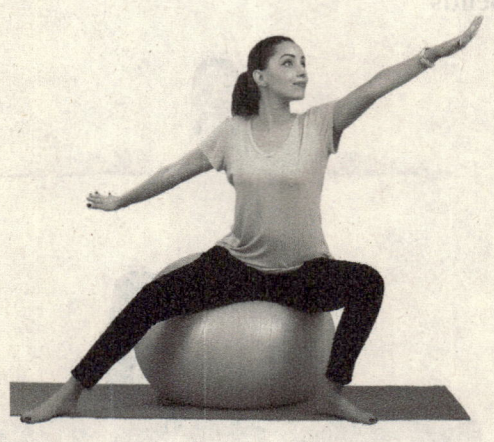

Keep consulting your antenatal therapist to help you with the exercises for labour. Do not perform or start any new exercises on your own.

Show your ultrasound reports to your antenatal therapist to understand the position of your baby. There are exercises to change the position of a breech baby. Your baby can be in a vertex/cephalic position, which is a head-down position required for a natural delivery, or a breech position—a feet-down position.

Continue all your breathing exercises. Remember your goal is to have a natural labour and you have to prepare your body for it. Do not exercise if you feel too low, weak or feverish. Wait for your body to recover.

You may also start hypnobirthing sessions to teach your body relaxation during labour for a natural delivery. Hypnobirthing is a technique that is used to take control of your mind during labour to manage pain. There are sessions that one can undergo to learn this art. It is very popular in the US and the UK, but not yet popular and easily found in India.

Start charting your baby movements now. You must feel average movements around six–eight times in a day, especially after every meal. If you notice fewer or no movements or if there is any vaginal bleeding, please call up your obstetrician and inform her.

You will be ready to deliver any time as you reach your thirty-seventh week. Learn all the signs of labour that you need to watch out for. You know your labour has started when:

- You experience frequent intense contractions.
- Water bag leaks or bursts.

- There is blood coming out from your vagina.
- There is a thick mucus plug coming out of your vagina.
- Continuous backache that doesn't go away.

Immediately inform your ob–gyn. Make sure that your hospital bag is ready. You may ask for a preparation sheet from your hospital or your antenatal therapist. There is no need to panic when you start getting these symptoms. You are just going to look forward to welcoming and receiving your baby with a calm and relaxed body.

As your baby is delivered, enjoy her as you will feel that your preparation for nine months has been worthwhile. You might experience a mixed set of emotions. You might want to cry out of excitement and happiness.

---

### THIRD TRIMESTER

— Enjoy eating.
— Add a lot of fibre, and have salads and soups.
— Drink vegetable juice.
— Have different fruits.
— Add endurance exercises.
— Prepare for labour.
— Walk every day for at least thirty minutes.
— Watch out for any signs of labour.

# 13

# Prenatal Parenting and Bonding

Being a parent actually starts right from the time you plan to have a child. However, parenting is a big responsibility. Just having a child doesn't automatically make you an authority on it. To have a child and to be a good parent are two completely different things. But meaningful parenting takes time and requires sacrifices and some conscious life decisions.

Are you a responsible adult? Can you take care of yourself, or of your partner? Because you sure as heck have to be responsible for your children provided you want them to grow up as conscientious, sensitive persons. You must identify your negative habits and get rid of them. If you have an unhealthy lifestyle marked by regular partying, smoking, frequent consumption of booze and drugs, a poor sleep cycle, anger issues, a sedentary job, among others, you need to seriously consider making some dramatic changes before deciding to bring a child into this world.

You must also assess your relationship with your partner. The signs aren't good if it is characterized by a sense of modern urban isolation, where you stay together and yet occupy different worlds, where you lie on the same bed and instead of talking to each other scroll mechanically on your phones. You must spend quality time with each other. If you're working and are too busy, you must find time. You cannot not communicate with each other over long periods of time. Communication gaps strain a relationship and can lead to frequent fights. Make sure that you go out for coffee once a week. If something is bothering you, discuss it with your partner. Encourage them to do the same. Try to listen to each other; be there for each other. One has to make adjustments and compromises for one's loved ones provided they don't erode one's sense of self. Understanding, helpful partners, tolerant of each other's differences are more likely to be great parents than two people in a strained relationship. If the problems are especially grave, a couple can approach a counsellor. It's important to create a warm, loving environment to raise a child.

Here are some tips that I would like to share with you and your partner as part of prenatal parenting:

- As a new mother, don't skip your supplements. As a partner, ensure that she doesn't.
- As a new mother, eat healthy and don't skip your meals. As a partner, make sure she has access to healthy food.
- As a new mother, don't drink or smoke. As a partner, do not do so around her.

- As a new mother, don't skip your prenatal check-ups. As a partner, accompany her on these visits; remind her about them.
- As a new mother, stay happy. As a partner, try to relieve her stress.
- As a couple, prepare for childbirth. Deliver as a couple and welcome your baby with an equal sense of responsibility.
- As a new mother, prepare yourself mentally to breastfeed your baby. As a partner, provide her maximum support for breastfeeding and give her as much help as possible.

> Don't just be a parent but be a good parent before your little one arrives.

## Prenatal Bonding Exercises

What your baby perceives during her time in the womb defines her. It is important to expose your baby to the right environment and feelings. She should feel relaxed, welcomed, loved and confident. The atmosphere at home should be conducive for her and not neurotic and turbulent. Work with your partner in trying to create an ideal atmosphere for raising your child.

These activities will help too:

- Write letters to your baby or keep a journal expressing your delight over your pregnancy. Share these with your child later when she grows up.

- Take pregnancy photographs.
- Record messages for your baby.
- Record siblings telling a story to the baby.
- Record messages from other members of the family.

## 14

# Sex during Pregnancy

It's not unusual to have concerns over sexual activity during pregnancy or how intercourse might affect the baby. As long as the pregnancy is proceeding normally, and both you and your partner want to, you can have sex as often as you like. Initially, for some of you, hormonal fluctuations, fatigue and nausea may affect your sexual drive. During the second trimester, increased blood flow to the sexual organs and breasts may rekindle your desires. But by the third trimester, weight gain, backaches and other symptoms may once again dampen your enthusiasm for sex. However, every couple is different. Consider what's best for the two of you.

As long as you and your partner are comfortable, most sexual positions are okay during pregnancy. As the baby grows inside your womb, experiment to find out what works best. Instead of the missionary position, trying having sex sideways or from behind. Let your mood and body understand what you want. Would you like to have sex or is the thought of it enough to make you uncomfortable? Your comfort zone is very important. Talk to your partner about it. Don't be hesitant.

Sexually transmitted infections may harm your baby. Use a condom to prevent such risks.

If you are not willing to have sex, it can be very distressing for your partner. Let them know that it won't be this way forever. There is more to a relationship than sex. Cuddling, kissing and giving each other a massage may seem more desirable.

**For Partners:** Try to understand it from the perspective of the mother-to-be. Is she eyeing the mound of laundry while you are trying to seduce her? Consider relieving some of the stressors around her so she has more energy to respond to your advances. Is she always tired at night? Then prefer mornings or a lazy afternoon when she feels up to it.

Try to understand the changes that her body is going through and be sensitive. Remember, thoughtfulness begets thoughtfulness, and if you respect her feelings, she may decide that she's not so averse to yours after all.

You can maintain intimacy in a number of ways. Stay connected during the day with short phone calls, emails or text messages. Spend a few quiet minutes with each other before the day begins or before going to sleep. When you are ready to have sex, take it slow.

You must prioritize your expecting partner's demands over yours—whether she is up for it or not.

Check with her ob–gyn if sexual activity is safe for her.

There is intimacy beyond sex. Expressing love, affection and care can make you and your partner feel complete in each other's arms as you look forward to the arrival of your baby. Let the comfort of the woman be more important. Be more understanding.

# 15

# Babymoon Time

Most upper-middle-class urban couples today choose
to holiday at the end of the second trimester. You
may travel if your ob–gyn lets you and provided you and
your partner will take adequate safety measures during
the trip.

## Travel by Air

Generally, airlines allow pregnant women to fly till their
thirtieth week but some have different rules. So check
before booking your tickets.

- Avoid long-distance flights. Choose a destination
  that's not too far away.
- You should choose a seat with extra leg space.
- Ensure that you are wearing your seat belt at all times
  to avoid abrupt jerks in case of bad weather.
- Drink lots of fluids during the flight.

- Keep doing your ankle exercises.
- Don't hold your urine for too long.

Once you land and check into the hotel, raise your feet by placing a pillow underneath them for a while; rest before heading out. A warm bath is extremely relaxing. Do find out the nearest hospital to the hotel in case of an emergency. You should actually keep this in mind while booking the hotel.

## Travel by Car

Avoid long drives as we don't want any bumpy roads to make you uncomfortable. Place your legs straight on the back seat or sit in the passenger seat with the seat belt on. Adjust the seat according to your comfort. Keep a pillow under your feet. Avoid non-stop driving for more than three hours. Take a break to do some walking to maintain your blood circulation and empty your bladder in a washroom.

Even if you can't leave the city due to some reason, you should still go for a holiday. You can maybe check into some nice hotel or a nearby resort and have a weekend getaway with your partner.

Holidaying in pregnancy during the safe period actually helps in bringing you and your partner closer; you can bond well with the baby too. It is an excellent relaxation method.

# 16

# Women Facing Challenges in Conceiving

## The Preconception Phase

There are lots of women who find it difficult to conceive due to various reasons. For example, polycystic ovarian disease or PCOD is a common reason that makes it difficult to conceive. PCOD is a condition in which the ovary enlarges and small cysts form on its outer edges due to hormonal imbalances. However, lifestyle modifications can help women overcome this disorder, along with other medical or fertility treatments.

Here are some lifestyle modifications for women who have issues with conceiving:

## Have Lots of Sex

Although it might be difficult to have sex regularly if you have a busy work schedule, it's not impossible. Try different things like massages or aroma therapy to rekindle more interest. As far as sexual positions are concerned, the missionary one is the best in helping sperms travel up the vagina. If you are married and live with your in-laws, plan weekend getaways to enjoy some much-needed intimacy and great sex. Your partner must avoid masturbation. Try to make them understand the fertile period of your cycle. The day on which you periods starts is day one. Your fertile period is from the seventh day till the fourteenth, of course, that is if you have a twenty-eight-day cycle. During this period, you should have sex frequently to increase your chances of conceiving.

## Watch Your Diet

Unhealthy food can lead to weight gain, which may further cause hormonal imbalance. Avoid starchy food, fried stuff and sweets. Take in a lot of antioxidants. They are found naturally in fruits, nuts and salads.

## Watch Your Weight

Too much weight can affect hormonal secretions in women. Hormonal imbalances can make you vulnerable to diabetes, insulin resistance, PCOD, thyroid and other diseases. Such conditions affect fertility. Try doing cardio exercises to lose those extra kilos.

## Sufficient Intake of Vitamin B$_{12}$

Vitamin B$_{12}$ supplements help in the better development of the baby's brain. It also prevents neural tube defects in the baby, the risk of which is pronounced if you have conceived at an advanced age. The older you get, the more difficult it is to conceive while the chances of chromosomal abnormality in the baby is higher.

## Cut down on Alcohol, Quit Smoking and Say No to Drugs

In women, alcohol reduces immunity, overloads the liver, slows down the brain, affects microbiomes in the body and hormonal levels as well, which can lead to fertility problems. In men, it leads to a reduced sperm count and sometimes erectile issues or the inability to ejaculate during sex. Reduce your alcohol intake to improve your chances of conception. In fact, I suggest you go for a detox and take a break from alcohol. This applies to both men and women.

Smoking, even passive, can affect the ovaries and the sperm count in both women and men. Drugs can lead to infertility. Avoid them.

Along with these things, you need to keep the following in mind too:

- You should also avoid stress. Studies have shown that too much stress can make one infertile. Try to relax. You can practise the various techniques and therapies mentioned in the earlier chapters. Go for holidays with your partner and try to stay happy and maintain a positive outlook towards life. I also recommend counselling sessions. They are very beneficial and provide the much-needed emotional support.

- Keep consulting your gynaecologist. She will screen you for hormonal levels and medical conditions that can affect fertility or lead to challenges in conceiving.
- Yoga sessions for couples might increase intimacy between your partner and you.
- Massages are helpful. A good head massage will help you relax and unwind. Foot massages are good for women who have irregular periods. The pressure points in the sole of the foot stimulate the uterine muscles, which improves blood circulation to the uterus and is also relaxing. Go for a foot massage when you near your ovulation phase, which is mostly between the tenth and fourteenth days of your cycle. You may also use ovulation kits that are available over the counter.

If you have failed to conceive even after trying over a year, you may need to see a fertility expert. She will guide you with the infertility treatments that are possible, depending upon the one that you may require.

## 17

# Breast Care in Pregnancy

Some of you may feel an increase in your breasts' size from the second trimester onwards and tenderness in them in the third trimester. It is important to take care of your breasts. You must keep them clean. Wash them nicely with warm water while taking a shower. In your third trimester, start doing massages with olive oil, especially from the thirty-second week onwards. I advise my patients to massage three–four times a day—before taking a shower, after the shower, once in the evening and at bedtime. This will prevent stretch marks and prepare the breasts for lactation by enhancing blood circulation.

## How to Do Massages

- Massage the left breast with your right hand and the right with the left in a circular pattern while putting pressure with your palm.
- Ten times clockwise followed by ten times anticlockwise.

- Then use both your hands to do upward strokes on the breast. Ten times on each breast.
- No downward direction to be used. Also no nipple massage to be done before the thirty-seventh week.

## Are Your Nipples Ready to Breastfeed?

You can assess the shape of your nipples towards the end of your third trimester. Some of you may feel that you have flat or inverted nipples. There are certain massage techniques that help in improving the shape of the nipples near the end of your pregnancy. You must consult your ob–gyn if can't figure out their shape.

## Wear the Right Bra

You must wear the right-sized bra. You might experience some itching around the breasts during the course of your pregnancy. Keep applying lotion. Avoid tightly padded underwired bras, especially in your third trimester, as they can make you feel uncomfortable and breathless. Avoid sleeping without a bra as it will cause more sagging and pain in the breasts. You may wear a comfortable sports bra at night if you find it more convenient.

You might experience some leaking or discharge from the nipples. Clean them regularly.

Also, preparation for breastfeeding is very important. Breast toning exercises must be performed. Breast toning can be done by doing wall push-ups, dumb-bell exercises for the chest (not more than 2 kg recommended) or using theraband.

## Pre-delivery Diet Tips for Breastfeeding Preparation

Add the following to your diet, apart from drinking lots of fluids, from the thirtieth week onwards:

- Coconut.
- Two teaspoons of flaxseeds.
- Ginger or garlic.
- Fennel.
- Methi.

# 18

# Precious Pregnancy

If you had been struggling to get pregnant or had to undergo many fertility treatments, or if you have a history of multiple abortions and miscarriages, then your ob–gyn would tell you to be cautious during your current pregnancy. Don't get scared; but you need to pay a lot of attention to your health and that of your baby's.

Gymming and swimming are a strict no-no.

Try to stay active if your ob–gyn allows you to in case no bed rest is advised.

If you work for twelve hours and spend a lot of time in commuting, you might be asked to quit or go on maternity leave early. You might feel depressed if you have to stop working for a while. But try to cheer up thinking that you will soon be welcoming a new member in your family. If you have been trying to conceive for a long time, no happiness can match the one that you will get after discovering that you're finally pregnant.

Keep a proper check on your baby's growth. Make sure you do not compromise on your diet, if at all any limitation is discovered in the growth of the baby or her weight gain. Be regular with all your tests and scans.

There are higher chances of having a pre-term baby in some cases and your ob–gyn might decide to deliver the baby early through a C-section if required. This happens when your baby is not growing well inside your uterus despite medicines, diet and supplements. In this situation, the baby might be kept under observation in the neonatal intensive care unit (NICU) for a few days. Remember that our aim is to ensure good health of your baby and not just the mode of delivery. If you do have a C-section, take sufficient care of yourself. Do core exercises as and when allowed by your therapist to strengthen your abdominal muscles that are cut during the surgery. Consult your postnatal therapist after a month of delivering the child and get your abdomen assessed. Certain exercises can help you heal faster.

Also, mothers get very worried when the baby is kept in the NICU. Make sure you visit the NICU whenever allowed and try to give your own milk for the baby.

# 19

# Labour Time

## Are You Thinking Right?

When you find your mind buzzing with a million thoughts as you approach your eighth month, remember to stay (a) positive, (b) practise meditation and (c) talk to your partner, friend or doctor to dispel your fears.

## What Happens in Labour?

You'll have mixed feelings when your labour starts. You'll be nervous and excited. Take deep breaths to get a grip on yourself and once in the labour room, keep asking the nurses about the status of your labour. You will feel less anxious when you know what's going on around you.

Most patients I meet are just worried about getting the baby out. You must understand that labour is a long process and giving birth is just a part of it (a major one, of course).

## Stages of Labour—Stage One

This first stage is further divided into three parts: (a) early labour, (b) active labour and (c) transition phase.

### a)  Early Labour

You contractions will be very mild and less frequent. You will be put on the cardiotocography (CTG) machine for monitoring the baby's heartbeats, and on some IV fluids. You might be given an enema to empty your bowels. So you will be visiting the loo frequently. Then your cervix will start dilating.

*Let nature take its role and do what it has to with your body to let your baby come out in a natural way, which has been happening since centuries.*

Just focus on deep breathing every time you get a contraction. They might last for around ten hours. Try to distract yourself by reading a book, listening to music or talking to a family member or your partner. You can also walk around. Remember, this is just the initial part. Don't panic. The more relaxed your body the more will your uterus contract naturally in pushing the baby out.

### b)  Active Labour

As your contractions get more frequent, stronger and intense, you'll move into the next level—active labour. Great news: we know that your cervix is dilating well and your baby is almost ready to come out. Stronger contractions are a good sign that your labour is on the right track.

Focus on deep breathing, followed by huffing and puffing when the contractions are too intense and back to inhaling deeply as they fade. The timing of the contractions is important to know if the labour is progressing or not. Urinate every one hour or as required. Your cervix will open up to 7 cm.

Here are some quick tips for you and your partner to refer to before you enter the labour room:

## Breathing for Labour

If you have been religiously practising deep breathing throughout your pregnancy, you will now be able to easily inhale for 7–10 seconds and exhale for 7–10 seconds as well. Remember to concentrate on your abdomen movement. This will help you as the contractions get stronger.

## Timing of Contractions

The timing of the contractions will help you take control of your breathing as they strike. Let your partner time them and maintain a chart. If a contraction lasts for forty seconds, try to inhale and exhale four times before the second one strikes.

## Change Breathing if Needed

As the contractions get more intense, you need to experiment with your deep breathing. You can do a position mentioned in the next few pages and focus on your breathing. Even then if don't get any relief, switch to huffing and puffing.

## Huff and Puff

Intersperse long deep breaths with short ones. If one contraction lasts for 60 seconds, do deep breathing for the first 15 seconds. As the contraction starts peaking, switch to quickly taking in a breath and exhaling for 15–20 seconds. Follow this by deep breathing again as the contraction starts fading. Relax yourself, wipe your face with a cold towel and take a few sips of water.

If this doesn't help as the labour progresses, you can try panting during the contractions. Panting breathing is rapid inhalation and exhalation through the mouth as if you have had a long run.

## Ice Chips

Sucking ice chips also helps in labour. You may carry some or ask for some in case they are available in the hospital.

## Labour Massages

Massages in the lower back, arms and feet can help reduce pain during labour.

## Empty Your Bladder

Urinate every one hour. You may not feel the pressure in your bladder but will be able to pass urine when you try.

## Track Your Cervical Opening

Your nurses or doctor will come and check your dilation a few times. Keep asking them about the progress to get an idea about how much more time it will take.

## Don't Stick to the Bed (If the doctor lets you)

Changing positions will help speed up cervical dilation and descent of the baby.

Aroma therapy is also a good idea. It will help you relax for a natural birth.

But in case you feel that you cannot bear the pain at all, you can opt for epidural anaesthesia. The anaesthetist will come and help you with an epidural to reduce your pain.

## c) Transitional Labour

As you move towards the end of active labour marked by multiple internal check-ups, you will now enter the third part. Ask your nurses after each vaginal examination about the cervical opening. This will give you an idea about how much more time it could take and help prepare yourself mentally.

This is the shortest phase lasting up to forty minutes to an hour or so. Remember, the breathing method will help you to cope with this stage as well. Your cervix will open between 7 and 10 cm.

## Different Positions in Labour

Lying flat on your back throughout labour will not help you unless it is medically important for you and your baby. Speak to your obstetrician regarding the different positions you would like to try in labour and with the help of your partner and the labour room nurses try them. It will ease the contractions and help in the faster opening of the cervix.

### Ball

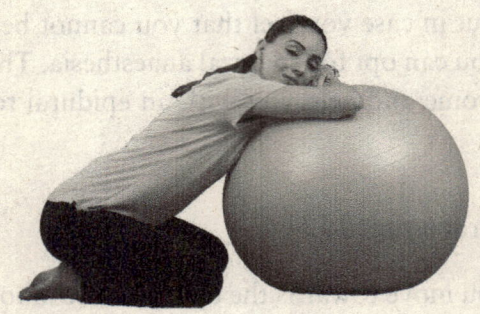

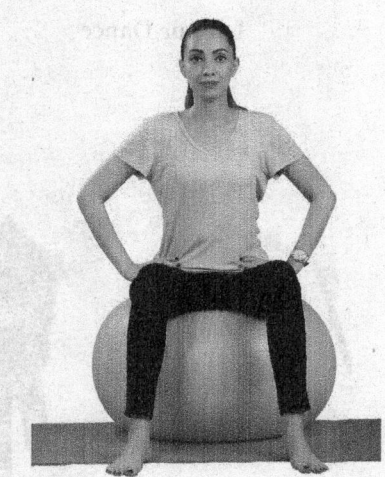

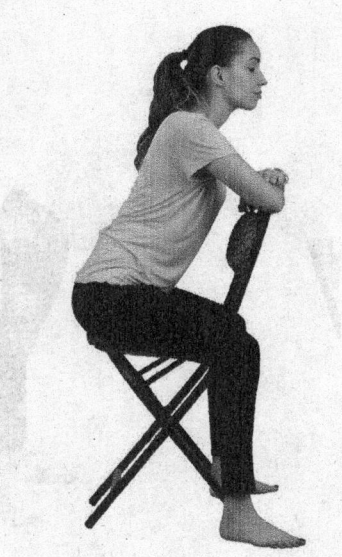

## Labour Dance

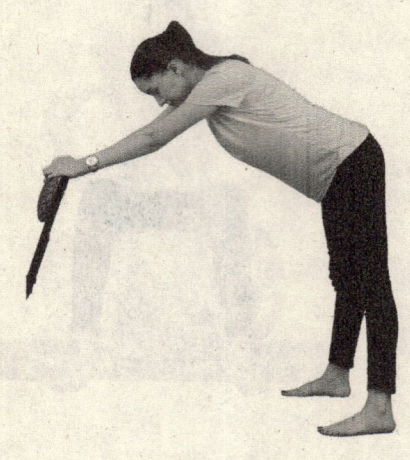

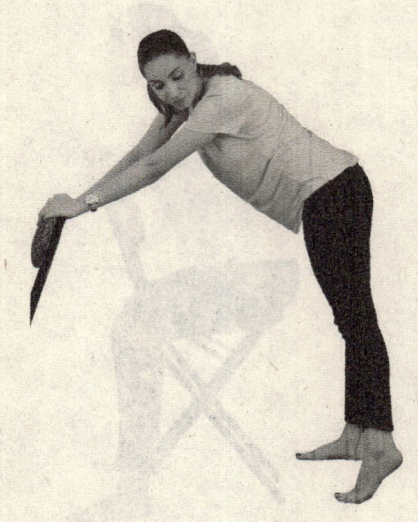

## Squatting

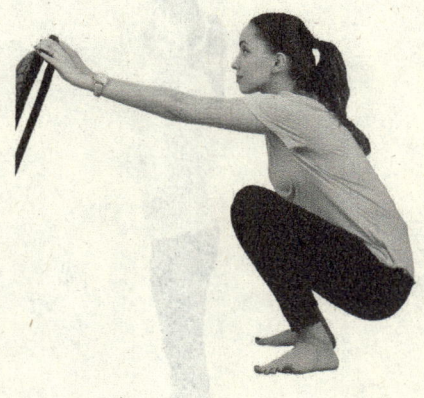

## Chair Lunge

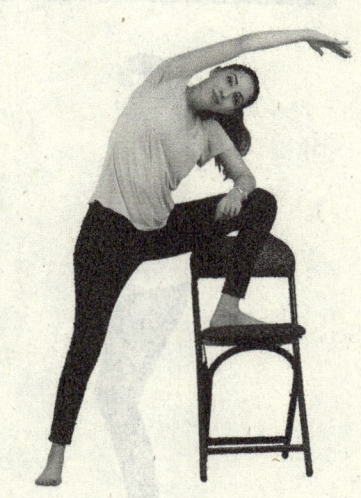

## Pelvic Tilts in Labour

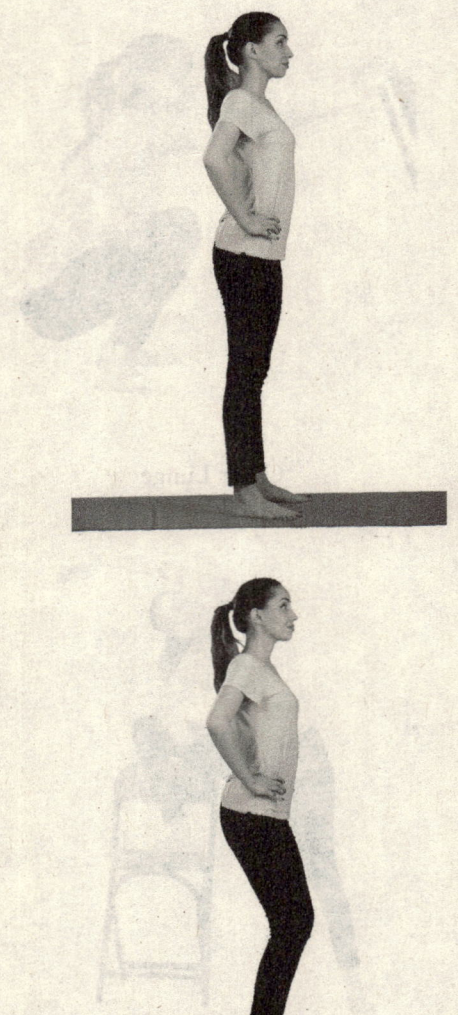

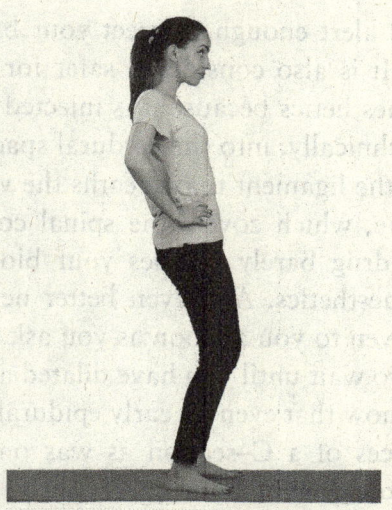

## Epidural/Pain Block

Epidural anaesthesia helps in reducing your pain. The anaesthetist's team will be informed; they will come and do a quick assessment and discuss your case with your ob–gyn. A decision will be taken based on the status of your labour and its progression. An epidural is generally not required in stage two as the anaesthesia can affect your ability to push. Its dosage and duration will be decided by the anaesthetist.

Almost two-thirds of labouring women delivering in hospitals prefer an epidural. The major reasons for its surge in popularity are its: (a) relative safety (only a small amount of medication is needed to achieve the desired effect), (b) ease of administration and (c) patient-friendly results (local pain relief in the lower part of the body allows you to be awake during the birth and alert enough to greet your baby immediately after it). It is also considered safer for your baby than other anaesthetics because it is injected directly into the spine (technically, into the epidural space that is located between the ligament that sheaths the vertebrae and the membrane, which covers the spinal cord). This means that the drug barely reaches your bloodstream unlike other anaesthetics. And even better news—an epidural can be given to you as soon as you ask for one. There is no need to wait until you have dilated a certain amount. Studies show that even an early epidural doesn't increase the chances of a C–section as was once believed, nor does it slow down labour significantly.

Here is what you can expect if you are given an epidural:

- Before the epidural is administered, an IV of fluids is started.
- Your lower and mid-back are wiped with an antiseptic solution and a small area on the back is numbed with a local anaesthetic.
- A large needle is pushed into the numbed area, which is the epidural space of the spine, usually while you are lying on your side or sitting up and leaning over a table or being supported by your partner. Some women feel a little pressure when the needle is inserted. Others feel a tingling sensation as the needle finds the correct spot. If you are lucky, you might not feel a thing while the epidural is being administered. Compared to the pain of the contractions, any discomfort caused by the needle is likely to be minimal.

- The needle is removed, leaving a fine flexible catheter tube in place. The tube is taped to your back so you can move. Three to five minutes following the initial dose the nerves of the uterus begin to numb. Usually after ten minutes you will begin to feel the full effect. The medication will numb the nerves in the entire lower part of the body, making it hard to feel any contractions at all.

- Your blood pressure will be checked frequently to make sure it's not dropping too low. IV fluids and lying on your side will help counteract a drop in blood pressure.

- Because an epidural is sometimes associated with the slowing of the foetal heartbeat, continuous foetal monitoring is usually required as well. Though such monitoring limits your movements somewhat, it allows your ob–gyn to monitor the baby's heartbeats and allows you to see the frequency and intensity of your contractions.

## Are You Ready to Push?

### Stage Two

Once you have dilated about 8 cm, you enter the second stage.

This is when you are asked to push out the baby. Remember, you need stamina to push. So conserve your energy in stage one with a lot of deep breathing. You will be asked to push when you feel a contraction. Take a deep breath, place your chin on your chest and hold your breath as you push (not more than 5–10 seconds) and then exhale through your mouth. Repeat if the contraction is still there or wait for the next contraction. Remember, small frequent pushes will give you more energy than one long push. Your partner can motivate you to push. Or do as your ob–gyn instructs you.

Try to stay positive; think about meeting the baby in a few hours. You must be relaxed.

You baby will take two steps forward and one step back. Your ob–gyn will inform you when she can see the head coming out. Just tell yourself that you are doing a great job and in a matter of minutes will complete a great task of delivering naturally. And you could be telling your success story of having a natural childbirth to your friends and motivating them to do so as well.

As you breathe, imagine that your vaginal muscles are opening up like a bud. Relax them as you breathe to make it easier for your baby to come out. If you tighten them, it will be difficult for the baby to come out. Remember that your jaw and vaginal muscles work in sync. If your clench your teeth or tighten your jaw, your vaginal muscles will automatically tighten. So focus on relaxing your jaw muscles and your face and exhale, loosening your vagina.

## Episiotomy

This is a para midline incision that is given to make the cervical opening bigger for the baby to come out.

Your ob–gyn might give you an episiotomy if required. Many patients panic thinking of getting an incision in the perianal area. But think about how easier it will be to push when the cervical opening becomes wider. Discuss with your ob–gyn if you want to add it to your birth plan. Try to access more information on it.

In episiotomy, you will get an injection of local pain relief before the cut. You may not need it in case you have already been given an epidural anaesthesia, or if your perineum is thinned and already numb from the pressure of your baby's head during crowning. Your ob–gyn will then take surgical scissors and make either a median, midline or mediolateral incision. After delivery, the cut will be stitched.

You will be advised to take some measures for the faster healing of your episiotomy stitches and to prevent any issues. Discuss this with your ob–gyn.

## Stage Three or Placenta Expulsion

Once the baby comes out, she will be placed on your abdomen and after a few minutes the placenta will be removed. You may be asked to push some more, if required.

You will hear your baby's cry and feel her skin against yours. This skin-to-skin contact is very beneficial for your baby. Ask for it in case it's not practised by your ob–gyn. Let that moment fill you with a sense of contentment for having had a successful natural birthing experience. Let it be preserved as a memory of success for your future.

However, during the entire process of natural childbirth, if at all the ob–gyn feels that there is any risk involved that demands an immediate Caesarean, then let her take that decision. Eventually, it's your and your baby's safety that is of paramount importance.

# 20

# Role of Birthing Partner or Husband

You need to prepare your partner for labour too. They can do a lot to make the labour easier, trust me! I have seen excellent results. You need to take your partner for Lamaze classes or make them meet your antenatal therapist, who will train them.

- As mentioned in last chapter, your partner needs to record the timing of the contractions. Ask them to carry a watch to the labour room and time the duration along with the frequency of the contractions.
- They will help you with the various positions and in walking around.
- They need to keep motivating you by telling you that you are fine and very soon the baby will arrive. And also that they love you a lot.
- They need to give you few sips of water whenever you need it.

- They need to keep wiping your face with a wet wipe as you might sweat a lot during labour, or cover you with a blanket if you feel cold.
- They need to remind you to take deep breaths as you get contractions.
- They need to play relaxing music and keep you distracted.
- They need to let you feel that you are not alone and that they are trying to be a part of it.
- They need to give you massages in labour when you want.
- Most important: They should not faint!

You can teach them the deep breathing exercises too as they might find them useful in the labour room.

Remember the final outcome: your baby will enjoy the feeling of being welcomed to the world as her parents prepare for her arrival.

> Be there for your partner as your baby is about to arrive. Let your baby know that you were a part of not just creating her, but also a part of her arrival.

# 21

## The Magic of Skin-to-Skin

The best place for your baby right after birth is on your skin and not in another person's arms. This skin-to-skin contact is also known as 'kangaroo care', because the natural warmth, protection and nutrition that a mother's body offers to her newborn is like the safe haven that a baby kangaroo enjoys in its mother's pouch.

After giving birth, your deflated abdomen becomes a nest of loose skin for your baby. The skin-to-skin contact helps in the natural regulation of your baby's heart rate and body temperature. It also helps her establish regular breathing patterns and sustain high, stable blood sugar levels. Exposure to the natural bacteria on your skin during the first hours reduces her risk of developing illness from germs in the environment. Newborns that lie on their mothers' abdomens after birth cry very little. Compare this with the often-upset babies that are examined and warmed in a warmer across the room or in the hospital nursery. It makes sense that babies respond well to touch. For forty weeks, she has been in constant contact with her mother's body. So when she is kept close to her mother's body after delivery, she feels safer and more secure.

Skin-to-skin contact can also facilitate breastfeeding. It helps in initiating the breast-crawl as well. When a newborn is placed on her mother's abdomen, in time she can make her way to her mother's breasts and actually latch on by herself. The baby is helped by the familiar smell of amniotic fluid on her hands, the smell and warmth of her mother's skin, the sound of her voice, and the 'target' of her darkened nipples.

This contact can also benefit you by keeping your oxytocin levels high. After giving birth, your uterus is the size of a grapefruit. In the hours and days that follow, contractions are needed to help shrink it to its normal pear size. Oxytocin levels are very high as your baby moves through your birth canal and remain high as you and your newborn first touch each other, stare into each other's eyes and breastfeed. The high levels of oxytocin keep your uterus contracted to reduce bleeding. This hormone also helps in being calm and responsive. In the days following birth, it wards off postnatal depression, continues to keep your uterus contracted and speeds up healing.

While lying against your skin, the baby's hand and head movements stimulate the release of additional oxytocin and endorphins, increasing milk production and keeping you and your baby calm and relaxed. Endorphins have been called nature's narcotic. When our bodies work hard, and when we feel secure, warm and loved, endorphin levels rise. Endorphins do more than block pain reception—in the initial moments after giving birth—they help accelerate a mother's ability to bond with her baby. Endorphin levels are especially high twenty minutes after giving birth, and are strongly present in breast milk. Immediate breastfeeding helps in giving a soothing effect to the baby and she can sleep better.

For all its physical and emotional benefits, skin-to-skin contact should be a carefully protected routine. During this intimate time, mothers become acutely aware of their newborn's needs and who is touching the baby and what's being done to her. Neither the mother nor the newborn misses a beat in the first two hours when left together, and others should trust them to follow each other's lead. The baby and mother will know when it is time for feeding; when it is time for comforting; when it is time for exploring.

To make sure you and your baby are given time for skin-to-skin contact, request that she is placed on your bare abdomen or chest right after birth, with a warmed receiving blanket laid over both of you and a cap on her damp head to help keep the warmth in.

If you give birth in a hospital, protocol may lead staff to suggest that you let them care for your baby in the nursery so you can sleep better. Make no mistake—giving birth is hard work and rest and sleep are important in the first couple of days. Without rest, a mother's exhaustion may lead to sickness, sadness, or feelings of being overwhelmed. Her tired, stressed out behaviour may make the baby cranky as she picks up on her mother's signals. To be a calm, rested caregiver, it's important that you sleep and rest, but that is actually easier in close physical contact with your baby. Studies show that mothers whose babies stay in nurseries don't necessarily sleep more or any better.[5] In fact, mothers and babies who stay together without any separation rest better. You may sleep more peacefully knowing that your baby is next to you. You are there to make sure she stays warm and you can immediately respond to her cries. During breastfeeding, high levels of prolactin and oxytocin actually help you relax and sometimes even doze off during the feedings.

Rooming in allows the baby and mother to rehearse the cues and responses that help with important developments—the mother can learn her baby's cues and needs more quickly, which means the baby can trust that her messages will get responses. This means that breastfeeding will have a better start as well. When your newborn awakens hungry with you holding her or just a step away, she sends signals that you have learned to recognize, and you put her to the breast well before she cries.

I strongly recommend that the mother and the baby sleep with each other after delivery. When the baby has fallen asleep after the breastfeeding session, keep her close to your body. It helps in continuing closeness. Also, the baby feels more secure and will sleep well. Even better, you can turn sideways and let her sleep close to your breast, which is also known as breast sleeping.

# 22

# Skin and Hair Care in Pregnancy

Every woman is different and so is her skin. No two women will experience the same skin changes during pregnancy. While some might be blessed enough to enjoy flawless, glowing skin in their third trimester, others will go through less-desired changes.

Skin pigmentation is a very common complaint in pregnancy, which is most common during the third trimester. The reason is hormonal changes. I always tell my patients that skin care in pregnancy is mandatory to prevent skin problems.

Let vitamin C and sunscreen be your skin's best friends in pregnancy. Vitamin C will help retain your original skin colour and the sunscreen will save the pigmented skin from harmful rays of the sun.

Remember that a lot of vitamin D is required during pregnancy. However, its absorption gets blocked by sunscreens. Avoid putting sunscreen on your arms and legs and sit in the sun for at least thirty minutes daily for vitamin D absorption. Don't forget to cover the face.

Let some vitamin D go directly into the bump—uncover the abdomen if possible and sun it as well.

Consult a dermatologist if you need help in choosing the right sunscreen. Regular cleansing, toning and moisturizing are a must. Clean the face with a mild, chemical-free face cleanser, followed by a toner. You may opt for a vitamin C-based toner. Use aloe vera-based moisturizers if possible.

A homemade serum—a few drops of almond oil, glycerine and two teaspoons of lemon juice—can be applied at night to prevent pigmentation and skin darkening on the face. Apply it with a cotton ball after cleansing, toning and moisturizing your face. Apply on your neck as well. You will see excellent results.

Face pack therapies can be really effective in preventing skin pigmentation that usually occurs in some women due to hormonal changes. Prepare a face pack at home with *besan*, haldi, lemon juice and aloe vera. Make a paste and apply it on your face, let it dry and then wash your face with cold water. Apply some rose water or a toner. Follow this with a moisturizer and a sunscreen if you are stepping out. You should do this once a week.

Stretch marks are the most common skin complaint of pregnant women. You cannot not get them when you are expecting. Most pregnant women develop pinkish or reddish (sometimes purplish), slightly indented, sometimes itchy streaks on breasts, hips and abdomen. Stretch marks are caused by tiny tears in the supporting layers of tissue under your skin as they become stretched to their limit. Expectant moms who have good elastic skin tone (because they inherited it and/or earned it through years of excellent nutrition and exercises) may slip through several pregnancies without a single telltale mark. If your mother sailed through her pregnancy with the smoothness of her skin intact, chances are you will too. I really wish there was a magic wand to make them go away. But dry skin is always more prone to stretch marks and itching than a well-moisturized skin. So keep your skin hydrated. The best feedback that I have got is from women who used coconut oil. You can apply it twice a day. Also apply vitamin E and cocoa butter-based lotions around the belly, breast and hips as these are the areas that stretch the most in pregnancy. My favourite is Palmer's cocoa butter lotion. You can also apply a calamine lotion if the itching becomes troublesome. But if at all it starts to give you sleepless nights, inform your obstetrician as it could indicate a raised liver function test level.

Excess weight gain will stretch your skin even more. Keep a check on it. Regular antenatal yoga and exercises will help in toning your muscles. Drink lots of fluids to stay hydrated. Eat right. Avocado, coconut water, lemon juice, almonds and walnuts will take care of not just your skin but your hair too.

## Hair Care

Hair fall is another very common pregnancy-related issue. Use a mild *amla* or Indian gooseberry hair cleanser every other day to wash your hair. Massage your hair with amla, or olive and almond oil for around thirty minutes before washing your hair for better results. Some women's hair might become more lustrous due to hormonal changes.

Avoid colouring, rebonding and other hair treatments from a salon during pregnancy. I allow my patients to colour their hair only if they have grey hair as it can get depressing, especially with pronounced mood swings. Don't colour your hair in the first trimester.

Avoid hair sprays as they contain too many harsh chemicals. Try to keep it as natural as possible. Simply let your hair loose and enjoy.

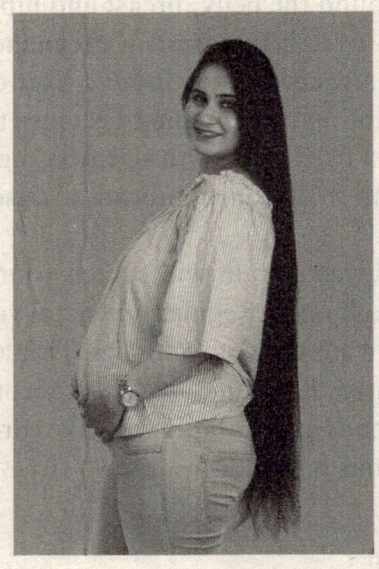

Don't tie your hair too tightly and do not let it become too oily as oil attracts more dirt on the scalp. In case of dandruff, use an anti-dandruff shampoo after consulting your dermatologist. You may apply some lemon juice and aloe vera gel in your hair before shampooing. A diet comprising vitamin $B_{12}$, iron and vitamin E will help in taking care of your hair.

# 23

# Shopping List Before Your Baby Arrives

For the mother:

- Nursing gowns
- Nursing bra
- Maternity sanitary pads
- Breast pads
- Feeding pillow
- Breast pump (optional; can be bought by working moms later)

For the baby:

- Cradle (whether to use one or not is a personal choice)
- Romper (multiple sets)
- Mittens
- Booties
- Socks
- Caps
- Baby blankets

- Diapers
- Cotton nappies
- Wrapping sheets
- Swaddling sheets
- Burping cloth
- Bibs
- Sweaters or warm lowers if it is winter
- Bodysuits
- Baby wipes
- Car seat
- Bath tub
- Diaper dispenser
- A baby bag

The list is endless. But depending on your budget and after discussing with your paediatrician, choose baby skincare products that can be used safely.

# 24

# Dental Care in Pregnancy

Dental care in pregnancy is an important aspect of maintaining good hygiene during this phase. Oral-cavity infections can possibly spread through blood circulation into your baby. Therefore, dental care remains an important aspect of pregnancy wellness. Many women say that their grandparents tell them not to use a toothbrush during pregnancy as their teeth would become loose. But brushing has to be done during pregnancy although tooth mobility can be affected to a certain extent.

Due to frequent acidity and recurrent vomiting, the acidic environment of the oral cavity may disturb the normal pH of the mouth. In this situation, dental caries may develop. Also, many women develop cravings for sweets and chocolates and often get midnight munchies, which further increase the risk of developing dental caries. You must visit a dentist in your second trimester for a routine check-up.

## Gingivitis

Bleeding from the gums is also a common problem during pregnancy. This again can be due to hormonal changes. Hence, rinse your mouth after every meal and have lots of vitamin C-rich sources such as oranges, lemon, etc.

Gingival infections can lead to elevated levels of inflammatory markers that occur as a response to the inflammation. This can be found in the amniotic fluid as well during pregnancy, which in turn increases the risk of a premature labour or low-birth weight.

In case any dental treatment is required, it should be avoided during the first trimester. You must inform your dentist about your pregnancy.

# 25

# Stem Cell Banking

The innovative concept of stem cells provides you with the once-in-a-lifetime opportunity to gift your child good health for the future by preserving her umbilical cord stem cells at the time of birth. Your child's umbilical cord is loaded with stem cells. These cells have the potential to treat certain critical ailments and can protect your child in the future if required.

Stem cells are 'master' cells that act as building blocks of the body to regenerate and turn into the cells that form all tissues, organs and systems in the human body. They are undifferentiated, 'blank' cells that do not yet have a specific function. Characteristically, stem cells have a high capacity for self-renewal.

Stem cell banking is a simple procedure. You have to enrol for it with a stem cell bank while you are pregnant and ideally a couple of weeks before delivery. Upon enrolment, you will receive a collection kit that will contain all the material and relevant information for you and your doctor.

Your ob–gyn or other staff will collect the cord blood and the cord tissue from the umbilical cord immediately after you give birth. The entire process takes less than ten minutes. Once the cord blood and cord tissue are collected, they will be transferred to the processing facility of the stem cell bank through a designated courier for testing, processing and storage. The stem cells are harvested from the cord blood and cord tissue and are preserved at the cryogenic storage facility.

Opting for stem cell banking is totally a personal choice. You should do some more research before you get convinced to go ahead with it. You can get in touch with stem cell banks and they will give you a home presentation about how the stem cell collection works and its scientific approach. They will also share with you the list of ailments that can be treated and the ones that have been so far treated by the use of stem cells from their bank.

## 26

# Pregnancy and Work

Most of my patients are working women. If you develop complications, you might be told to continue working at your own risk. Even if there are no complications and your ob–gyn has given you a green signal, you still need to see if your body allows you to continue working. But remember, pregnancy doesn't mean that you have to discontinue working. But maintaining your fitness and wellness will help your body work for as long as possible during this phase. Most of my patients have been able to work till their ninth month with the help of fitness and wellness classes.

## Commuting to Your Workplace

You must have a look at the distance between your home and office. How long does it take you to reach your workplace after taking traffic into consideration? In a long-duration journey that might last for forty minutes or an hour, you could have to pee. Then what will you do? If you have an eight-hour-long shift, along with which you spend around two hours travelling, then you are technically 11–12 hours outside your home. Such a routine may cause physical discomfort at a certain point in your pregnancy. You could be more stressed out, have pains and aches as you wouldn't be getting enough rest. It might be difficult to follow a proper diet, access clean washrooms, which might lead to you holding your urine for long, something that is not at all advisable during pregnancy. Time and distance plays an important role in choosing to continue your job. Your mode of commuting also matters. A bumpy commute is not recommended. Avoid metro rides if your health doesn't allow you. You may discuss this with your ob–gyn and partner.

Don't try to be a super woman. You must listen to your body. Never push the body beyond its capacity in pregnancy. You should try discussing with your boss or seniors at work if the company can support you in any way. Do not be afraid to start such discussions. Remember that pregnancy is your right as a woman and you do not need to let it be a reason for not finding solutions to your problems even if it means involving your boss.

## Stress at Work

Stressful work characterized by constant deadlines can aggravate health issues in pregnancy. Like I have said earlier, exercising, meditation and yoga will help manage stress. You can do the breathing exercises and meditation even at your workplace. Or you can take a day off or short leave to refresh yourself. You can plan a weekend getaway with your partner to relax and pamper yourself.

But if in spite of all these measures you continue feeling burned out, prioritize your body over work. Sit with your ob–gyn and ask her if you should continue working or if there is some other solution.

## Posture at Work

If you are a lecturer or a teacher and stand most of the time at work, you must demand a chair during pregnancy. Standing for long durations can aggravate pregnancy-related issues such as varicose veins, swelling in legs, cramps, pain in the feet.

Regular blood circulation needs to be maintained. Poor blood circulation can cause dizziness and you just cannot afford a fall in pregnancy. So sit down with your boss and explain this to them.

Important precautionary measures are necessary not just in standing jobs but for sitting ones as well. Most jobs nowadays require women to sit in one place for a long time. If you have such a job, you need to take extra care of your posture as pregnancy leads to many changes in your natural spine alignment. Your muscles tighten during pregnancy leading to more pain and less flexibility. Also, your spine curvature changes due to the baby bump. So you have to consciously try to maintain the right posture.

Exercises that involve postural correction, such as stretching exercises, will really help you. I always tell my patients that it is mandatory to maintain fitness in pregnancy. The spine goes for a toss later when you have to breastfeed your baby frequently, making any pain and posture worse. So spine care has to start right now. Prevention is the whole purpose of this book. So try to sit or walk tall always and do specific exercises regularly.

You must do basic stretches every three hours in office. These include neck stretches, leg stretches, side bends, arm stretches, etc. Try to take a break and go for a small walk every two hours.

Go fill your water bottle and remember to drink two glasses of water every hour. The more you drink water, the more you will have to pee, which will automatically make you leave your chair and walk. Drinking adequate water will also prevent urine infections and keep the baby healthy.

Keep practising Kegels while sitting in your chair. But make sure that you have emptied your bladder. Walk for 5–10 minutes during your lunch break after having a meal.

Sit with your feet raised on a foot rest. Gravity will cause pooling of blood in the legs and worsen the blood circulation. So you have to keep your feet raised above the ground level while you remain seated in office or perhaps even at home. Try to adjust the level of your desk and chair according to your height to make it ergonomically comfortable for you, making sure there is enough space for your baby bump and the table.

## Sitting Posture

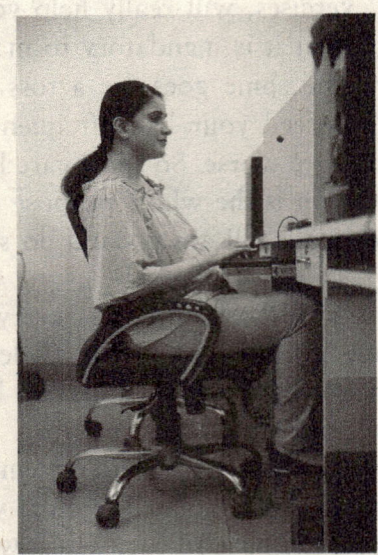

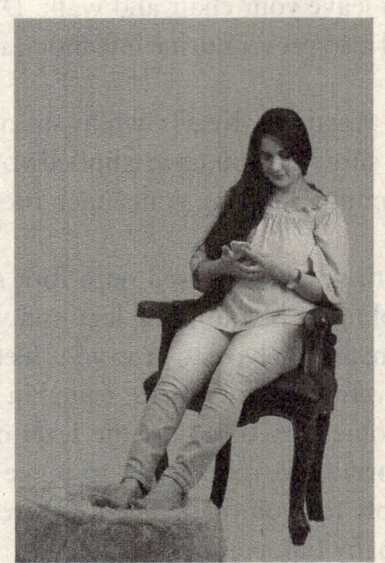

## Lifting an Object from Floor

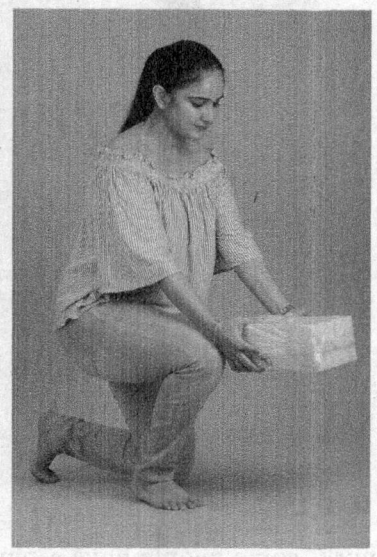

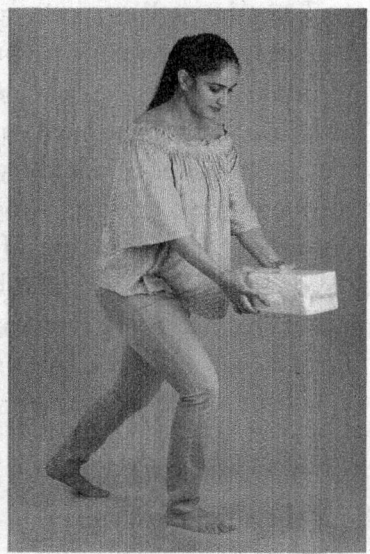

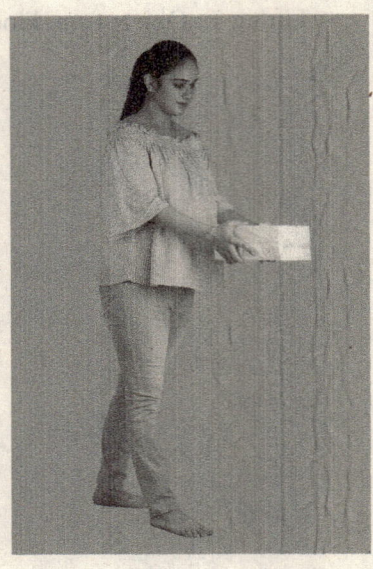

While at work, some people have a tendency to drink a lot of coffee to keep themselves awake when they feel low on energy. During your pregnancy, you have to restrict your caffeine intake. Excessive caffeine can restrict the growth of the baby. So as mentioned earlier, do not have more than one cup of coffee or tea every day. Remember, chocolates also contain caffeine. Along with tea and coffee, also look out for the amount of chocolate you're consuming. Pregnancy cravings should be enjoyed, but in the right amount. An excess of everything is bad. If you have milk in the form of cold coffee, switch to normal cold milk or a fruit shake or protein shake—these are much healthier options for your baby. Depending upon your medical condition, discuss with your ob–gyn or dietitian about the amount of milk you should take.

## Snacking at Work

You must always carry something to munch in your purse to office. Never step out of the house without it. Refer to the healthy snacks mentioned earlier in the book. Remember to have small, frequent and healthy meals throughout the day. Try not to eat at your office canteen if you're not too sure about the conditions in which the food is prepared. It is preferable to carry your lunch from home. Avoid food with preservatives. Also, avoid packaged juices as they contain both preservatives and added sugar.

## Clothing at Work

Wear loose and comfortable clothing. Avoid tight clothes.

## Footwear at Work

Do not wear heels to work. It will aggravate your backache and leg pain. Wear shoes or flats.

# 27

# Tips for Your Partner

It is always heart-warming to see partners taking out time for antenatal visits. You must involve yourself as much as possible in the pregnancy.

Here are some tips for you: practise some breathing exercises and meditation for at least ten minutes with your partner in the morning before going to work. You must create some time. It's for your baby.

Give your partner a call while you are at work. Let her feel that you care even when you are not around. Ask her if she has had her medicines and meals properly. Try to understand that pregnancy can make her feel nauseated and she might try to skip her meals. Show concern, encourage her to eat on time.

As you come back from office, get her fresh coconut water. Sit down with her for some time before you change your clothes. Ask her how her day went.

Take her out on weekends for dinner or for a movie and/or shopping. You may prepare the shopping list in the third trimester and head out for that.

Sit down with her and keep a record of her visits to the doctor. Try to accompany her for antenatal check-ups and scans. Let her feel that you are equally excited about the baby. If you are not able to accompany her and miss a visit, make sure you ask her what the ob–gyn said. Show your complete involvement. Keep yourself updated about the baby's status.

Cope with her mood swings. It won't be easy but that's the challenge. Accept it and face it. Blame the hormones, don't blame her. Just cuddle her and love her.

Give her your maximum emotional and physical support; give a helping hand at home; prioritize her wants over yours.

If you are married and your family compels her to follow some traditional customs during the pregnancy, make sure that she does only those things that are scientifically good for the baby and herself. Don't force her. Most such customs are myths. Let her discuss with her ob–gyn first.

Do a survey with her for choosing the birthing place. Visit a few places with her; let her see where she feels comfortable. Hygiene, medical service, quality service, experts are some of the factors that must be kept in mind while choosing the right place. Don't let your family pressurize her into delivering at the same hospital where your mother delivered you. Make use of new facilities. There are many special maternity centres that have specialized experts and services for labour and baby care. Choose one of them. They also have antenatal classes, breastfeeding support, etc., which other hospitals and nursing homes generally don't offer.

Having a baby will increase your expenses. So sit with her and make a budget for the pregnancy, a shopping list, plan to hire maids, etc. Make your baby the priority; start saving for her. All this is part of parenthood. Our parents have also worked hard in trying to give us the best. You might have to cut down on other areas for a while if your pocket doesn't allow some expenses, but remember to prioritize the comfort of your partner and baby over your wants.

Take out time for shopping for the hospital bag with your partner. This is not a one-day task. It can take some days. Visit a few stores, do some online research before deciding upon the brands. There are many available in the market, but take a decision based on your budget, of course. Ask your doctor for suggestions.

## Did You Know?

### Sympathy Symptoms

Feeling curiously . . . pregnant? As many as half, or even more of expectant dads suffer from some degree of sympathetic pregnancy during their partners' gestation.[6] Symptoms include nausea and vomiting, abdominal pain, appetite changes, weight gain, food cravings, constipation, leg cramps, dizziness, fatigue and mood swings.

Any number of emotions in your psyche can trigger these symptoms, from sympathy (you wish to feel her pain, and so you do), anxiety (you are stressed out about the pregnancy or about becoming a parent) to jealousy (she's under the spotlight and you want to share it). But there's more to sympathy symptoms than just sympathy. In fact, there are actually physical factors in play. Believe it or not, your partner's female hormones aren't the only ones surging these days. Research shows that pregnancy and the postpartum period step up a father's supply too. Although you and many others like you aren't churning enough hormones to grow breasts, you might produce enough to grow a little belly or salivate at the sight of your favourite burger or run to the fridge for a midnight pickle fest.

These hormonal fluctuations aren't random or a sign of Mother Nature's twisted sense of humour. They are designed to get you in touch with your nurturing side. This not only prepares you for diaper changing, but helps you to cope with the changes that both of you are facing now. These hormonal shifts make it easier for you to channel those sometimes uncomfortable feelings into productive pursuits. Apply your sympathy in cooking dinner; work through your anxieties by talking them out with your partner and friends.

These symptoms will soon disappear after delivery. Some others may crop up in the postpartum period. And don't stress out if you don't have a single sick or achy day during your partner's pregnancy. Not suffering from morning sickness or putting on weight doesn't mean that you don't empathize and identify with your partner, or that you are not destined for nurturing. You just have to find other ways of expressing your feelings.

You can also practise breathing exercises and follow a healthy diet to stay fit during this phase! ☺

## Be There After Delivery

The very best way to start your new life as a parent is to be at home with your family. So if it's possible and financially feasible, consider taking off as much time as you can right after your partner gives birth—some companies give paternity leave, or you could go on an extended leave. If possible, you can even consider working part-time or from home. Should none of these possibilities prove practical, and given job responsibilities, maximize the time that you are at home. Learn to say no to overtime, early or late meetings, and business trips that can be put off or passed off. Especially in the postpartum period when your partner is still recovering from labour, try to do more than your share of household chores and baby care when you are at home. Keep in mind that no matter how physically or emotionally stressful your occupation is, there is no more demanding a job than caring for a newborn.

Make bonding with your newborn a priority, but don't forget to devote some time to nurturing your partner as well. Pamper her when at home and let her know that you are thinking of her when you are at work. Call her often to offer support and empathy, surprise her with flowers or take her out to her favourite restaurant.

# 28

# The Fourth Trimester

**M**otherhood is the natural end to pregnancy. However, it is not easy and comes with a lot of responsibilities. Your priorities change. Coping with the changes that come after giving birth can be taxing. So you must prepare yourself mentally for it.

Many mothers don't like to breastfeed their babies. Usually, such women prefer bottle-feeding as their presence is not required. Maybe other women you know claimed that their babies gained more weight after having formula feeds? Or maybe advertisements selling nutrition products have subliminally influenced your decision? These and many other reasons could have affected your choice. But try to rise above the cacophony of these various factors and think clearly. When you decide to have a child, you choose to go to the best ob–gyn, the best hospital, buy the best baby products. So why compromise on your baby's feed?

A doctor will always advise you to breastfeed as it has innumerable health benefits for you and your baby.

Even WHO recommends exclusive breastfeeding for the first six months. However, in case you have a specific medical condition, your doctor might tell you to switch to another form of feeding. But let that decision be taken by your doctor and you. I recommend all my patients to make a decision about feeding during the third trimester itself so they can mentally prepare themselves for it and learn the various ways to do it. Discuss with your antenatal or postnatal expert if you have any queries or apprehensions.

As a part of my antenatal sessions, I even prepare my patients for breastfeeding. The initial few weeks will be challenging. Your milk production will take up to five days to get a good flow; your baby will take a few days to set a feeding pattern and you may take a while to learn how to feed. The learning comes best with practice and the right guidance. You could face issues like breast pain, nipple pain, heaviness that extends up to the arm pits, etc. But don't let these reasons come between your breasts and your baby's wish to breastfeed. Your baby would demand feeding frequently, which is absolutely normal.

Sit down with a lactation consultant—this is a must if you are a new mother—and take some counselling sessions with her. You must learn the right holding techniques, latching and unlatching techniques, hunger cues, feeding positions and burping methods. These are the basics that play a big role in breastfeeding the right way. I educate my patients on these aspects even before they deliver the baby so that they know what to do from day one. If you have not been able to learn these techniques from an expert during your pregnancy, make sure you learn them from the expert in the hospital before you get discharged so that you feel confident while feeding your baby at home.

Your baby is hungry when she starts opening her mouth and moving her neck from left to right, or tries eating her own hand and then starts crying.

There are mainly four feeding positions—the cradle position, the cross-cradle position, the side-lying and the football.

## Right Latching

When the baby is placed on the abdomen of the mother immediately after delivery, she can smell her mother's breasts, which is similar to the amniotic fluid. This induces her to crawl towards the breasts. She will use her hands and feet to move up. This movement is called the breast crawl. I strongly recommend my patients to have the breast crawl as part of their birth plan and to ask their partners to ensure that the nurses assist in performing it after delivery.

While breastfeeding in order to stimulate the sense of smell, bring your nipple close to your baby's nose. Let the baby get the smell of your nipple, give her a few seconds and then slide it over her lips from her nose to her chin. Wait for her to open her mouth. If she doesn't, repeat the same process until she opens her mouth. While latching you have to ensure that not just the nipple but even the surrounding part—the areola—goes into the baby's mouth. This is the right way to latch and is a good way to prevent breast issues as you lactate.

Breast odour acts as a strong stimulus for the baby to reach the nipple. The smell mimics the odour of the amniotic fluid that was purposefully left on the baby's hand. Reaching out for the nipple indicates that the baby's sense of smell is well developed.[7]

The little finger is used to break the latch and then the breast is removed from the baby's mouth. Ensure that after each feed, correct burping is done. Place the baby on your shoulder and pat her back gently while holding her in an upright position. Sometimes babies can take a longer time to burp so keep them upright on your shoulders for at least 10–15 minutes if the burp is not audible.

Try to meet your lactation consultant within a week after your discharge to be sure that you have learnt it right. Also, discuss with her the challenges that you are facing with your feeding. If you are experiencing too much breast pain beyond seventy-two hours of delivery, you could be suffering from engorgement in the breast that needs to be treated. Breast engorgement happens when the milk is not being expelled properly, which results in pain and heaviness. It can lead to feeding difficulties for your baby. So it must be prevented. In this case, you need a breast massage with oil and hot fomentation. Also, the milk needs to be expressed.

## Crying Baby

Don't let your family influence your ideas on breastfeeding. Many mothers come to me saying that their babies are not getting enough milk as they are always crying. Firstly, as a mother you need to understand that you are the decision-maker. Secondly, as the mother you know best when your baby is hungry. Learn the hunger cues properly. Your baby will display these cues before she cries. In fact, she will cry only when you miss these cues. So make it a habit to respond to her cues before she starts bawling.

Also, the baby is not always hungry when she cries. She could be crying due to other reasons—feeling cranky or insecure, seeking attention, feeling too hot or cold, bored, or hurting somewhere. Remember that she can't speak as yet so crying is a way to express herself. Use the back of your fingers to touch her tummy and see if it is too hot or cold. Wrap her up and bring her close to your body if she's cold. She could just be seeking your attention. Lift her up and start walking or try to swing her in your arms. Also, check her diaper, it could be time to change it. You must understand this and explain it to your family as well. Involve your partner and family members in also taking responsibility of looking after her when she cries. Never let this be a reason to switch to formula feeds.

## Colicky Baby

Sometimes your baby may cry for up to three hours in a day continuously. If this happens, talk to the paediatrician. You baby could be having colic pain, which can cause a lot of stress to you and your partner as well. Ensure that proper burping is done after each feed. Make sure to feed the baby on each side too. Babies suck in a lot of air while feeding. Sometimes this air inside their bodies can cause colic pain as well. Burping helps in removing this excess air. Proper latching generally helps in reducing the chances of excess air going inside the baby. Please sit down with your paediatrician and explain the crying pattern to her. She will give you some tips. You need some help from her in case your baby has colic pain. Try to keep the baby in your arms. Colicky babies feel more comfortable when carried in the arms rather than being laid on the bed or in the cradle. Tummy massages can be helpful too but only light pressure should be applied.

## Postnatal Depression

It's absolutely fine to have emotional outbursts in the initial postnatal phase. There is so much new happening at this stage if you are a new mother—the excitement of having your baby in your arms, the uncertainty of fulfilling your role as a mother, family pressure, sleepless nights, crying baby, hormonal changes, feeding, cleaning and wiping the baby, etc.

Postnatal depression is very common after delivering the baby. But you can cope with it by keeping some things in mind. Try to motivate yourself; tell yourself that you are doing a great job as a mother and that every day you will learn something new to be a good mother.

But it may sometimes get worse, especially if there is lack of support from your partner or family, or if your baby is not doing well medically. You definitely need support in taking care of your child. If it's just you and your partner, then someone from your families need to stay with you for at least the first month after your child is born. Keep a domestic help if you can afford it. Again, don't try to be a super mother. If you feel severely depressed, please see a counsellor. It might make things better.

## After Pains

Your uterus will continue to have contractions. This is post-delivery pain, which you will experience for a few days as your uterus starts rising. Breastfeeding helps in aiding the rise of the uterus due to release of hormones. So you would experience some contractions during breastfeeding. It's absolutely normal. The pain won't make you go into labour again. ☺

## Lochia

Of course, there is blood loss at the time of delivery. You will continue losing some blood even after delivery for some days. This condition is called lochia. The quantity of blood loss varies from woman to woman. You have to use thick maternity pads in case of heavy bleeding to avoid staining your clothes. There is no fixed period for this bleeding. Make sure you eat well and continue your supplements if the ob–gyn advises you to do so in case of excessive or prolonged bleeding.

## Postnatal Check-ups

Make sure you go for all your check-ups advised by your ob–gyn. I advise my patients to at least visit the ob–gyn three–four times in case of a natural delivery, if not mentioned by your doctor. Also, most ob–gyns send their patients for a cervical cancer vaccination after childbirth. If you haven't had the vaccination earlier, make sure you talk about it with your ob–gyn, if she doesn't mention it.

## Does the Bump Still Show?

You will lose a few kilos after giving birth to your child and as the placenta is removed. But it won't be any visible difference. Don't freak out. Your bump may still be there. That's fine. You will lose some weight with breastfeeding. Exclusive breastfeeding helps you shed those extra kilos faster. Give at least four weeks to your body to recover and for you to get used to the presence of your baby. You could meet a dietitian after a month to start thinking of weight loss. But we don't want any crash diets to lose weight. It has to be healthy to prevent any deficiencies and weaknesses. Follow the right way. Of course, exercising plays a big role in toning your abdomen. You may start after four weeks in case of a natural delivery. Some exercises will be taught to you before you are discharged by the physiotherapist that will help you recover faster. Continue doing them at home for four weeks.

You should continue wearing maternity pants. Don't expect yourself to fit into regular clothes immediately. Let it be gradual and just make sure you are on the right track. You definitely don't want to put on weight after your delivery. So keep checking your weight every two weeks.

You should wear nursing gowns or nursing dresses that will make it easier for you to feed your baby. Comfort while breastfeeding is very important since you may have to do it for a long time. Discomfort is one of the reasons why mothers give up on breastfeeding early and easily.

## Disturbed Sleep Cycle

It will take time for you to have a fixed sleep cycle during the initial period. You have to stay up at nights, along with your partner and family members, for the baby. But remember, you need at least eight hours of sleep daily. The best thing to do is to try to sleep whenever the baby is sleeping. Normally, babies tend to have a fixed sleeping pattern from the third month onwards. However, your baby could be either a day sleeper or a night one. Avoid too much caffeine as some of it can pass on to your baby through breast milk.

## Contraception

It is ideally recommended to have a gap of at least two years between your first and second baby. However, it also depends on the mother's age. Discuss with your ob–gyn if you want to have another baby. But you must use some measure of contraception after delivery to avoid an unwanted pregnancy. Let your body recover first. Take your partner along with you when you discuss with your ob–gyn about contraception, let them also be counselled on this. Breastfeeding prevents pregnancy but is not a 100 per cent measure against it, so don't rely on it.

## When to Resume Sex

With the episiotomy and stitches, soreness and some after pains, mostly all women lose their libido for some time. Sex is the last thing on their minds as they are busy getting used to all the changes. Also, as women bleed for the first few days, sex could be painful. Breasts are sore due to breastfeeding for the first few days. But some men think that it is absolutely fine to resume intercourse after delivery. Talk to each other and discuss your comfort level and what your body allows you to do. Cuddling and kissing could be great as it also helps in overcoming postnatal depression.

## Baby Expenses

The list of things to buy for the baby will be never-ending. You will just finish off paying the hospital bills only to realize: 'Wow! That much to just have a baby!' So, plan your expenses. Spend wisely. You'll get gifts from friends, relatives and colleagues. You can maybe tell them your preferences, depending upon their budget. Don't be shy as this is a practical thing to do. Also, many a time people end up giving you things you already have. So no harm letting at least your close ones know what you have already bought.

# 29

# Early Parenting

When your baby arrives, you spend more time listening to and learning about her than you've ever done before. You focus all your attention on her; she has so much to teach you about caring for her. You learn more about parenting from each other than you can ever from any website. Try to be in as quiet a setting as possible when you're with your baby. It is difficult to learn the baby's behaviours in a setting with distractions.

Speaking of distractions, you will receive advice as never before from friends and family. Most of it is well-intentioned. But a lot is uninvited as well; some may hurt your feelings; others are plain misinformation.

Your relationship with your baby is unique, and together you are charting unknown waters. So when a friend tells you her secret for getting a baby to stop crying, or when your mother suggests that you put your baby on sleeping and eating schedules, you may need to turn a deaf ear.

When someone, particularly your mother or mother-in-law, gives you unsolicited advice on how to care for your baby, you may feel defensive, hurt, angry, judged or inferior. The elevated levels of hormones in your postpartum body may keep you on edge for a while. A comment that you may have shrugged off before can now be stinging. To help you deal with unwelcome advice, repeat the following to yourself—

- I have every reason to trust *myself* to care for my baby.
- I know my baby, and I am learning every day to listen to her.
- I am wise enough to understand her demands.
- I shall follow only what my doctor tells me and not what everyone else says.
- I shall trust the experience of my doctor for my baby.

At the same time, simply thank the person offering the advice and change the subject, or if they are determined to expound, excuse yourself politely.

## Parenting Your Baby—Hold Me, Feed Me, Love Me (Mommy, Don't Leave Me)

Nils Bergman, a public health physician, points out that although our babies are born with the skills and behaviour they need to grow and be healthy, they are the most immature of all mammals. As a result, they require a great deal of care, almost as if they were still in the womb. According to Dr Bergman, the mantra our babies chant is 'hold me, feed me, love me'. Keeping the baby close to you and responding to her needs quickly builds trust, empathy and affection. It also ensures that the baby will thrive physically and emotionally. Close, responsive, baby-led care is what nature intends for those first months of life. It might even be considered the golden rule for parenting.[8]

During your pregnancy when you caressed and spoke to your belly, you fostered loving attachments to your unborn child. When you insisted that she stay with you once born, you continued this feeling of closeness. And when she is at home, you have the opportunity to lovingly respond to her cues and signals, to her cries, and to things in her environment that might distress her. Just as your newborn thrives on touch in those first few hours, she will continue to flourish if you stay close and respond to her. This style of parenting will continue to decrease stress levels for you and your baby, helping her relax and sleep and grow and learn.

## Postnatal Massages for Mothers

Massages after delivery have been practised since ancient times in India. However, during those times the massages were done in very non-scientific ways. For example, the pressure applied during the massages was not according to the comfort of the mother; they were done by the *maalish-walis*, as they were called back then. They had no scientific knowledge or certifications and only learnt how to massage from their seniors.

Nonetheless, massages after delivery work as magic for new mothers. But when is the right time to start these postnatal massages, in natural deliveries and for those who've had a C-section? The answer depends on the part of the body that is to be massaged.

Some birthing centres in India offer foot massages after delivery. These massages have a therapeutic effect in case of pedal oedema. Post-delivery, many mothers have swelling and heaviness in their feet. This happens due to impaired blood circulation in the body. Massages help improve not only blood circulation in general, thereby reducing the swelling, but also around the uterus and the pelvic area as the pressure points in the soles are massaged. They are also a great way to pamper a new mother. These massages induce relaxation and relieve stress as a new mother struggles to adapt to the many changes happening in her body and in rearing the child.

In case your hospital or birthing centre does not offer foot massages, you could ask your partner or a family member to give you one on the second day after delivery. Aroma oils could be used or olive oil.

> Foot massages reduce stress levels after delivery that can help in a happier breastfeeding experience.

Massage the legs in an upward direction from ankle towards the knee. The downward direction should be avoided to reduce swelling in the feet. These massages help in reducing leg pain.

## Massages for the Core Region (Abdomen and the Lower Back Area Surrounding the Pelvic Region)

Massages done in this region will help in improving the blood circulation in this area. This should help in faster healing. However, ensure that the massage is being done with soft hands. Instruct the person giving you the massage or the maalish-wali to apply only light to moderate pressure that can be comfortably tolerated by your body.

## Shoulder and Neck Massages

As the breast size increases during pregnancy and while lactating, upper back pain is common. Lifting your newborn in your arms for feeding can lead to shoulder pain if feeding pillows are not used for support. It is important to maintain the right posture while feeding. Shoulder and upper back massages help in relaxing your shoulder and upper back muscles. Breast toning and arm and shoulder exercises are also important to prevent pain.

## Head Massages

Head massages are effective to induce relaxation and sleep. Light head massages also reduce the risk of postnatal depression.

> Stress affects breastfeeding too. Postnatal massages induce relaxation and help in better breastfeeding.

## When to Start Postnatal Massages

Foot massage, head massage, shoulder and neck massages with light and soft pressure can be commenced from the second day onwards for C-section mothers. For core region massages, wait until your ob–gyn gives you a green signal.

In case you've had a natural delivery, all the massages can be started with light pressure. This is how you should be massaged for the first seven days and gradually the pressure can be increased from light to moderate. Ensure that you are comfortable with the pressure. It should not cause discomfort.

> Head massages can help in improving sleep in case of a disturbed sleeping pattern.

Breast massages can be done on your own before a bath and before bedtime while you are lactating. The massage techniques have been mentioned earlier in the book. Regular massages prevent chances of pain or engorgement.

Remember, you need to take care of your own wellness too along with your baby's. However, please do not get too carried away and ignore the demands of your baby or your responsibilities as a new mother.

## Baby Massages

Generally, paediatricians in India recommend that you must wait till the umbilical cord stump falls off before starting baby massages.

Also, there are many products available in the market for massaging your baby. Remember, her skin is as new and delicate as a flower bud. Don't experiment with products; consult your paediatrician before using any product on your baby's skin. Olive oil massages are generally considered the best for your baby's skin. However, babies can be allergic to a skin product. In case rashes develop after any specific oil massage, discontinue usage of that product.

Make massaging as playful a time as possible. Keep talking to your baby; look into her eyes; play some music; hold her hands and feet to encourage limb movements as an exercise. Let her feel free to kick her legs and arms after the massage. It can be then followed by a warm bath. You may breastfeed your baby after that and she will doze off for a while.

Follow instructions of your paediatrician for baby massages.

# 30

# Your Little One's New World

Your baby will take her time to stretch out of the foetal position that she was in for so long. There's so much for you to see as your baby unfolds her fingers, arms, and the numerous creases in her skin. Her beautiful, tiny fingernails and toenails may let you spend hours in contemplation.

The biggest part of your newborn's body is her head. Labour and birth may have temporarily changed its shape or moulding, but it will look normal within a few days. She may have a blister on her head, a caput, which develops as her head presses against your cervix during labour. It will eventually disappear.

She has tiny ears; silky, slicked down hair, if she has hair; and if the lighting isn't too bright, wide-open eyes that seek you out. The puffiness in her face will decrease now that she's out of the watery womb. Increased hormone levels at birth have made her genitals swollen, but it will decrease as the levels get balanced.

Your newborn will probably keep her hands closed into little fists even when she's asleep. Her grasping reflex is so strong that you can help her pull herself into a sitting position. Even her little feet, with the toes lined up like peas in a pod, will try to grasp like hands when touched.

The following sections describe your baby's appearance, abilities and behaviour in more detail.

## Skin and Sense of Touch

While your baby was in the womb, your body made vernix—a creamy white, lanolin-like substance—to cover and protect her skin. She will be born covered in a little or a lot of vernix. Your baby's body may also still have lanugo—downy hair that covered her in the womb. It will disappear within a couple of days.

She spent the last forty weeks comfortably and safely immersed in the amniotic fluid and covered in vernix. After birth, there is no reason to wash away the vernix or the scent of the amniotic fluid. In fact, it's particularly important that the fluid's scent stays on your baby's hand so she can taste and smell it and connect the scent to the taste and scent of your skin. Once born, she can be patted dry with warm towels as she lies on your bare chest or abdomen. A lifetime of baths and showers, soaps and towels awaits her, but the first precious moments should be spent touching and connecting with you.

In the first couple of days after birth, your baby's skin and the whites of her eyes may take on a yellowish tinge. This colouring, called jaundice, is related to the bilirubin levels in her blood. Bilirubin is a pigment produced by the normal breakdown of the red blood cells in the liver, and it's discarded in the stool. The normal process of eating and excreting prevents bilirubin levels from becoming dangerously high.

Jaundice is common in babies because their livers are still developing and removing extra red blood cells needed for foetal circulation. The yellowish colour will fade away within a week or two as your baby eats more and her liver matures. A breastfed baby sometime stays yellow for a bit longer, but this condition is absolutely normal. If your breastfed baby is nursing well and gaining weight, there is no cause for concern.

To treat jaundice, some hospitals routinely place newborns under a special ultraviolet light to help break down the bilirubin in the skin. However, this procedure is rarely necessary. In fact, some experts now believe that jaundice may be a normal phenomenon in newborns. To prevent jaundice from becoming a problem, breastfeed your baby at least ten to twelve times a day. The extra feedings will help your baby excrete extra bilirubin in her stool. You might also expose your baby to sunlight. The ultraviolet rays work the same way as the hospital's artificial 'bili-lights'.

The skin is the body's largest sense organ, and babies thrive and develop best when their skin is touched. Not only does immediate and constant touching stimulate the production of growth hormones and aid the immune system, but it also helps establish better sleeping patterns and prevents distress.

In the weeks ahead, carry your baby against you or in a sling or a front carrier as often you can. The contact will let you both learn how to respond to each other's signals and needs. Consider giving your baby a daily massage to relax and quieten yourselves together. This applies to both you and your partner. Even they must spend a good amount of time carrying the baby in their arms or in a carrier bag while going out for a walk. The close contact with the other parent will strengthen their bond too. They must also give massages to the baby, after learning the right techniques, of course! Skin-to-skin contact, as mentioned in the earlier chapters, is very important for you and your baby.

Many families in India believe that the baby should not get too used to being carried around in the arms all the time. Many of my patients say that their in-laws or grandparents have told them so. Please understand that a newborn needs a lot of care and comfort. When the baby is carried around in the arms, she feels more comfortable and secure. This is especially important for colicky babies.

A few babies develop acne on their faces in the initial months. It could be due to various reasons—allergy to some product or cow's milk; coconut-oil massages on the head or face, etc. Once the reason has been identified, get rid of it immediately. In case the acne persists as the baby grows, consult your paediatrician to rule out these factors. Also, let your paediatrician check for any other causes. Remember, all babies are different.

## Mouth, Voice and the Sense of Taste (Oral Stimulation)

Your baby's mouth may look like a beautiful little rosebud. But from this perfect, tiny orifice, she will emit a mighty cry. At birth, some babies cry more than others and some require more attention in response to their cries than others. You may have seen a mother insert her pinkie finger into the baby's mouth to settle down the little one. This action meets two needs—to be held and to suck.

The sucking and rooting reflexes are your baby's most important survival tools. Immediately after birth, she may begin to nudge (the rooting reflex) towards your nipples, which throughout pregnancy have darkened into targets that she can see easily. Your baby will suck them in response to stress or fear, as well as for comfort and nutrition. The first few hours of breastfeeding will transmit colostrum into her little body. Continued sucking will eventually produce milk and help contract your uterus, as mentioned earlier. Some babies are ready to breastfeed right away after birth. Some may need a little more time, choosing to nurse a little more sedately. If your baby is a strong nurser, a little blister can form on the inside of her upper lip.

Your baby's taste buds were already developing when she was just eight weeks or so into gestation. While in the womb, she tasted the spices, flavours and chemicals that you ate and absorbed and passed on to her through the placenta. During the first few months, she will respond positively to only sweet flavours—your breast milk is sweet to taste. Paediatricians no longer allow honey to be given to the baby at the time of birth. It can cause botulinum infections in newborns. Only colostrum is allowed to be given at the time of birth. The clinical presentation of a botulinum infection can vary from mild hypotonia to severe bulbar paralysis and to sudden infant death. The typical symptoms include constipation, followed by lethargy, listlessness, poor feeding, ptosis, dysphagia, and loss of head control, hypotonia, visual problems, dry mouth and generalized weakness. Botulism can lead to paralysis lasting for days and weeks, and in some cases to respiratory failure. Fever is usually absent. Once the diagnosis is clinically suspected, single-fibre electromyography (EMG) studies help; it typically reveals increased jitter and block.

The spores of BoNT-producing clostridia are widespread in soil, dust and aquatic sediments and infants are considered to be repeatedly exposed. Despite this, infantile botulism is a rare disease and some other factor, such as a disturbance of the infant gut flora, is thought to be providing a window of opportunity for any spores present to germinate, colonize and produce toxin. For most cases of infantile botulism, the source of spores is never identified and it is assumed that they are swallowed from the environment. However, honey is a dietary reservoir of *C botulinum* spores for which there is both microbiological and epidemiological evidence. In order to minimize the risk of infantile botulism, it is recommended not to give honey to less than one-year-old. There is a widespread practice of administering honey or 'ghutti' (an herbal concoction mixed with honey) as a prelacteal feed to newborn babies among Asian families. In a study conducted in Pakistan, 15.6 per cent of babies received honey as prelacteal feeds, often influenced by the elders in

the family. A similar study from India reported most
of the grandmothers and mothers believed in early
feeding of newborn, within two hours of delivery,
by giving prelacteal feeds such as ghutti and honey.[9]

## Eyes and Sense of Sight

At birth a newborn's eyes often appear red and puffy,
and there may be broken blood vessels in the eyeballs,
caused by pressure exerted on them during birth or by
the drops or ointment she may have received after being
born. The eye colour changes. Permanent colour won't
develop for about six months in case of green, blue and
grey eye-coloured babies. Some can produce tears from
birth, but most don't for six weeks or so.

The dark, beautiful orbs peering out from your
newborn's face can see objects at close range (eight to ten
inches). Research shows that babies can recognize their
mothers in as little as four hours after birth. Your baby
can even respond to your facial expressions, especially
when you are within eight to ten inches of her face.
Studies confirm that movement attracts babies' sight
and newborns prefer curved shapes over straight ones;
patterns in contrasting colours over plain ones, and
ordered patterns over random ones. And they find the
human face the most attractive thing to look at.

Eye contact indicates that your baby's neurological
development is progressing normally. A baby who makes
eye contact is showing that she knows what a face is and
understands that facial expressions can indicate how a
person is feeling. It also makes bonding stronger between

the parent and the child as it shows you that your baby knows who you are and how important you are in her life.

The moment when your baby's eyes first meet your own is one of the most heart-warming milestones of infancy. New parents who are eagerly waiting for this day often wonder when their baby will reach this level of development. While all babies develop differently, most do meet developmental milestones, such as eye contact, on a fairly similar schedule. Being a little early or late usually doesn't impact overall development or change the bond that blossoms between the parent and the child when this moment finally arrives.

Parents typically notice the first direct eye contact from their baby at around six to eight weeks. However, there is a much wider range that is still considered normal, and some perfectly normal, healthy babies don't initiate eye contact until three months of age. Babies do recognize eye contact from parents as early as two days after birth, according to a 2002 study in the *Proceedings of the National Academy of Sciences*. The newborns in the study preferred to look at faces of people who were looking directly at them instead of those with an averted gaze.[10]

Your baby's alertness at birth allows for her first 'reading lesson', assuming no drugs were given during the birth process to dull her responses. As you and your baby gaze at each other, you are reading each other's cues, sending each other messages, making contact. Your baby may stare at you intently for a long period as she sorts through the surrounding stimuli. Or she may close her eyes, desiring a little more time before entering the bright, stimulating new environment. These hours of alert gazing send parents this important message: 'pay attention!'

## Ears and Sense of Hearing

Months before your baby's birth, she can hear your internal body sounds as well as the sounds of the outside world—voices, especially yours, rumbling vehicles, ringing bells, barking dogs and sounds that surround us every day. All that she hears from within is what she will recognize easily after birth. So try to surround yourself with sounds that are soothing and joyful for her even in your third trimester. Within the first hours of life, her tiny ears channel a great deal of information, helping her analyse and categorize the new surroundings. She will try to recognize the voice of her father too if she's been hearing it before birth.

Studies show that newborns prefer a live human voice over a recorded voice and an animated voice over an emotionally flat one. Babies also prefer to be looked at while spoken to. When you instinctively speak directly to your newborn in a gentle, high-pitched voice, she will listen and respond in recognition. She will turn her head to the source, open and brighten her eyes, and move her arms and legs.

I have noticed some mothers silently feeding their babies after delivery without talking or making eye contact. Don't do that. Talk to her while trying to breastfeed her in the initial few days. She will try to recognize and respond to your voice. Give her attention by talking to her when she is awake. She will respond by moving her hands and feet. And then try latching her on to the breast. Talk to her in a soft voice or sing in her ears when she cries. She will find soothing music very relaxing and it can help put her to sleep.

## Nose and Sense of Smell

At birth, your newborn's nose appears flat and broad. Her brain's olfactory (smell) centre forms very early in foetal development, so she is likely to have a sense of smell at birth. Her sense of smell and taste helps her reach your breast and nurse. Studies show that within a few days of birth, your baby can distinguish between the scent of your milk and skin odours. Certainly, your aroma is the most familiar and comforting for your baby—yet another reason to not wash away the amniotic fluid or vernix from her skin right after birth. It is also a good idea to wrap her in soft clothing that you have worn to let your smell comfort her.

## Behaviour

At birth, reactions to the new environment vary from baby to baby. If she isn't separated from you, she will likely pensively and inquisitively stare at her new surroundings for an hour or much longer. If she has been separated from you, she will probably become distressed as she seeks the comfort of your skin to reassure her that she can trust the new surroundings.

Your newborn may begin vocalizing right away, making little grunts or whimpering rhythmically while staring at her new world. It is as though she is waiting to hear some familiar, gentle and reassuring words and sounds that she can respond to. Or your baby may be more reserved, seeking the safety and comfort of your arms a bit longer before more actively engaging with her surroundings.

Researchers have observed several states in newborn behaviour.[11] Your baby's behaviour will follow a pattern that will develop at its own pace.

- **Quiet Alert State:** If any drugs given during labour and birth haven't dulled her responses, your baby's first hour is one of attentiveness and quiet inquisitiveness. She focuses all her energy in looking directly into your eyes and listening to surrounding voices. After this initial quiet alert state in the first hour of life, there are often few such prolonged periods over the next few days. Usually, briefer periods of curious, exploratory behaviour occur around feeding time. In the first week of life, the normal baby spends only 10 per cent of any twenty-four-hour period in this state.
- **Active Alert State:** During this state the baby is very different. She moves her arms and legs every two or three minutes, makes small sounds and looks around. These bursts of movements happen before feeding or when the baby is fussy. Play with her and prepare for breastfeeding.
- **Drowsy State:** The baby is still trying to open her eyes frequently while she feels sleepy. This state occurs right before your baby drifts off to sleep or right after

she wakes up. It's similar to how you feel right before you doze off on the couch, or just as you crawl out of bed in the morning in search of that first cup of coffee. In this state, your baby may continue to move a little as well as smile and frown.

- **Quiet Sleep State:** The baby can wake up with any disturbing sound in the room; try to maintain silence. She will often drift into this state at her mother's breast. This state is deep and peaceful, with regular breathing, closed eyes and few body movements.

- **Active Sleep State:** In this state your baby moves her eyes in sleep as well as her arms and legs; her breathing will speed up and she will display a variety of endearing expressions—goofy smiles, grimaces and frowns—in quick succession. She will tend to move or root around, as though trying to get closer to an edge or object. Babies generally move towards the warmth, sound and smell of their mother's body in bed before they settle into a quiet sleep. When she's waking up, she is usually coming out of active sleep. She will not wake up no matter how much you try to touch her and move her. Then we know she is definitely enjoying her beauty sleep and will wake up only when she wants to. Let her enjoy her sleep. You can also take a nap till then as your body demands rest too.

Just enjoy watching all these behaviour patterns of your baby and be patient. Remember, it is your patience that will keep you calm as you get adjusted to your new parenthood. Let her sleep peacefully. Avoid having too many relatives and guests in the room while you are still at the hospital. Both the mother and the baby should avoid disturbing sounds and loud noises. You need to ask guests to come one by one and speak softly.

# Afterword

In my career, I have encountered so many women who don't have access to the right information on taking care of oneself during pregnancy. As a result they often have complications or put themselves at high risk of developing some problems towards the end of gestation.

Pregnancy and menopause are the two transitional phases in a woman's life, apart from adolescence, when her body undergoes a tremendous number of hormonal changes that demand special attention. Every woman must take care of her health and her body, especially during these times.

During pregnancy, everyone worries about the baby's health even before she's born, but your body and health are precious too. One of the most important ways of taking care of your body is through prenatal exercises. Every pregnant woman must exercise during her pregnancy to stay fit and healthy, but only after checking with her ob–gyn as in some cases, such as low placenta and short-cervical length, exercising can lead to premature labour.

Also, eating right at this time is important. If you exercise and don't eat right, you can put yourself and your baby at risk.

Thinking right is another important point that expecting mothers should keep in mind. Do not get scared by the thought of a natural childbirth. Keep reminding yourself that you are going to prepare yourself and your partner/husband for it and will get rid of all your fears. Gain the right knowledge, get coached properly and happily look forward to having a natural childbirth.

The aim of my book is to make childbirth an easy and smooth process for expecting couples and to promote more natural deliveries in our country. Through this book, I also seek the support of other ob–gyns in our country to help me in this endeavour. Together we can succeed in spreading awareness about mother and child wellness as much as possible.

# Acknowledgements

Firstly, I'd like to thank God.

I was very keen on publishing with Penguin Random House India and Preeti Chaturvedi was a godsend who helped connect me to the right people there.

To my fantastic supporter and dear friend, Gurveen—who has shown continuous support and guided me with her ideas to make this book more appealing for the readers. Thank you for completing this book with me.

To Indrani—for making me love my own book even more with your fantastic editing.

To Rachna—hope to write more books with PRHI in the future.

To my mom—from whom I inherited my creative side and who inspired me to do something for all moms. You have always been a pillar of strength for me and supported me in all my dreams.

To dad—for letting me fly.

To my grandad—who was always proud of all my achievements. I wish you were here to see my book. I know this would have been your proudest moment.

To my sisters, Mansha and Mukta didi—for always celebrating my achievements with me.

To my mentor, Dr Suchitra N. Pandit—thank you, ma'am, for taking out time from your super busy schedule and helping me with this book. You are a wonderful woman and my role model.

To Dr R.K. Bali—for guiding me on the chapter on dentistry. You are a true inspiration to so many of us in our family. Thank you, Tayaji.

To my maternity model for this book, Prabhneet Kaur—thank you for letting me do a photoshoot with you. You look stunning and I adore you. I knew I wanted to shoot with you for my book when you used to come for my antenatal classes.

Thanks also to the people at Dipak Studios where I have done all the photoshoots for my book. Y'all are fantastic!

To my mentor at every stage of my career, Dr Ali Irani—thank you for holding my hand and guiding me to where I have reached now.

To Dr Alka Kriplani and Dr Anupam Sibal—who took out time to share their thoughts on *Birthing Naturally*. Thank you so much! Dr Sibal's book inspired me to become an author. Thank you, sir, for inspiring me to complete my book. Thank you, ma'am, for always being there whenever I needed you. You are doing great work for our country and I wish to learn so much from you.

Thank you Fortis Escorts, Faridabad, Apollo Cradle India, Birthright and Rainbow Children's Hospital for believing in me and giving me all the support to do great things for expecting mothers.

# Notes

1. https://www.ncbi.nlm.nih.gov/pubmed/1635490.
2. http://americanpregnancy.org/pregnancy-complications/pregnancy-induced-hypertension/.
3. Ballantyne, J.W. *Expectant Motherhood: Its Supervision and Hygiene.* London: Casell and Co., 1914.
4. Pathak, P.K., Abhishek Singh and S.V. Subramanian. *Economic inequalities in maternal health care: prenatal care and skilled birth attendance in India, 1992–2006,* 2010.
5. https://www.ncbi.nlm.nih.gov/pmc/articles/PMC1948089/.
6. https://www.ncbi.nlm.nih.gov/pmc/articles/PMC3628883/
7. https://www.ncbi.nlm.nih.gov/pmc/articles/PMC3647724/; Lothian, Judith and Charlotte DeVries. *The Official Lamaze Guide: Giving Birth with Confidence.* Minnetonka: Meadowbrook Press, 2005.
8. https://www.ncbi.nlm.nih.gov/pmc/articles/PMC3448763/.
9. Judith Lothian and Charlotte DeVries, *The Official Lamaze Guide.*
10. www.livestrong.com/article/494102-when-eye-contact-in-infant-develops/
11. Judith Lothian and Charlotte DeVries, *The Official Lamaze Guide.*

# About the Author

Dr Mahima Bakshi is a renowned woman and child/adolescent wellness expert in Delhi–NCR. After completing her bachelors in physiotherapy, she went on to undergo training in women's health under the guidance of Dr Ali Irani, president of Indian Association of Physiotherapists, in Mumbai. She was supported by the Federation of Obstetric and Gynaecological Societies (FOGSI) and received recognition for her contribution towards wellness for expecting mothers by Suchitra N. Pandit (head of obstetrics and gynaecology at Kokilaben Dhirubhai Ambani Hospital in Mumbai, and president of FOGSI, 2014–15). She has been trained in prenatal, perinatal, postnatal and lactation education. She has also studied family counselling and has done her certification in global adolescent health from University of Melbourne. She is currently pursuing an advanced PG certification in mother and child health.

Dr Bakshi has been upheld as an icon for women's empowerment and received awards from Union information and broadcasting minister Smriti Irani in support by Manav Rachna International University, the Ministry of Railways, Jiva Ayurveda and Rawal institutions. She is a social activist, and has been a health columnist for *Absolute India*, a Mumbai-based newspaper. Dr Bakshi is a familiar face on TV, being regularly interviewed by various channels such as CNN-News18, News X, etc., especially on International Yoga Day.

She has worked at Apollo Cradle Royale, Fortis Escorts, Faridabad, and Birthright and Rainbow Children's Hospital, New Delhi. She created and designed a mother and child wellness programme, Preggo, for Apollo Cradle. She is a strong supporter of breastfeeding and launched the first lactation clinic in Faridabad at Fortis Escorts Hospital to guide mothers on lactation challenges. Dr Bakshi also conducts workshops on adolescent health, believing that care for adolescents' health starts from the preconception stage, for Times of India NIE initiative in various schools in Delhi–NCR.